How To Win In The Youth Game: The Magic Of Plastic Surgery

HOW TO WIN IN THE YOUTH GAME: THE MAGIC OF PLASTIC SURGERY

by
Kurt Wagner, M.D.
and
Helen Gould

PRENTICE-HALL, INC., Englewood Cliffs, N.J.

How to Win in the Youth Game: The Magic of Plastic Surgery
Copyright ©1972 by *Kurt Wagner and Helen Gould*

Printed in the United States of America

Prentice-Hall International, Inc., London
Prentice-Hall of Australia, Pty. Ltd., North Sydney
Prentice-Hall of Canada, Ltd., Toronto
Prentice-Hall of India Private Ltd., New Delhi
Prentice-Hall of Japan, Inc., Tokyo

Library of Congress Cataloging in Publication Data

Wagner, Kurt
    How to win in the youth game.

    1. Surgery, Plastic. I. Gould, Helen
joint author. II. Title. [DNLM: 1. Surgery, Plastic
—Popular works. WO 600 W133h 1972]
RD119.W33   617'.95   72-4905
ISBN 0-13-441329-6

Foreword

THE CHARISMA of bare feet, generally dirty?

Or the ultimate world order in which man finally comes to learn how to live with himself?

While one is walking into the other, is our homogenized era creating a new breed of human?

Noise pollution (one of the fact-phrases we live with) tests claim that some young people may have already lost some of their high decibel hearing to some of the higher decibel sounds of music.

I believe that our central nervous systems are already undergoing a change in becoming tolerant of shock, violence, sonic booms, and the other cataclysms we are going through, from discothèques to jet disorientation. We have been going through more such changes in the last fifty years than in the whole previous history of man.

But is it the time of fulfillment, or the year zilch?

During no phase of man's time on the planet earth has he been so fascinated and intrigued by the promises of a seemingly limitless future—while faced with the possibility of no future at all.

In our present newly unzipped world, just as man seems about to lose his timeless hangups—is he going to lose everything along with them?

Is time growing shorter with the ticking of each second—or does an open stretch of realization lie ahead?

A doctor's entire life style is reconstruction, at the very opposite pole from destruction. In a time when, let alone what is happening to the people on it, our planet seems to be in the process of destroying itself, where is a doctor to find his own peculiar relationship to our growing, ubiquitous uncopemanship?

5

A plastic surgeon, perhaps of all men of medicine, goes beyond a concern with life to a concern with integrating life to its fullest capability.

The former euphemisms attached to the reasons for having plastic surgery have become "newphemisms." The accepted approach was that patients should be psyched out along with their surgery—to make sure they didn't want to improve themselves for the wrong reasons!

We come from this nasty suspicion to realize that plastic surgery is an adjunct to living, and should be used as such. If, indeed, psychiatry's purpose is to make one able to cope with life, then plastic surgery can be a kind of operative psychiatry in making an integrated life possible.

And a plastic surgeon is uniquely of this particular time—tied in now with the question and outlook that seem to have propelled us already into the twenty-first century.

Will it be the time when everyone will be beautiful and nobody will be old?

Will we be a planet of robots that do all the work, computers that do the thinking, and man himself a half-human, half-robot creation of technology?

Or will there *be* a planet?

Just as the individual man leaves part of his life behind him in stages, collective man is at the point in time where he is ready to move on to a new stage of his development.

The transition period is a tough one, especially when we cannot even be sure that we are going anywhere.

Young people are walking to India in search of themselves, among them the son of a movie superstar who owns one of the largest diamonds in the world. These young people are having experiences that blow holes in the mind.

Communication-alienation and confrontation are the new semantics between the straight world and the new one that youth wants to make.

While there seems to be a breakdown of conventions in all

6

directions, conventional thinking is actually what has broken down, so that we are breaking out of old, conditioned molds and trying to make new ones.

Youth believes the individual is a whole entity, not part of an entity. It is youth who is making new individualistic patterns of acceptance rather than following a code of morals within a framework existing since the time of Roman law and even twelve centuries before that.

Out of the uncopemanship of law enforcement, we may find the best possible solution—if laws have regulated our actions, we can come to regulate ourselves.

Youth requires a new world of morality and reality that it can believe in. The new morality is based on the truth about ourselves. It is youth who has at last come to see that it is not the match that starts the forest fire, but the man who holds the match.

And if it appears that youth is to take over in an age of anti-reason in a world where the supreme importance is to be young, who are the idols of youth?

Boston Brahmin Buckminster Fuller, who draws the diagram of the future; anthropologist Margaret Mead, who sees the age as a revolution-evolution she digs with accord; writer Henry Miller who has projected, and is still projecting, a few choice words about almost everything; and that great guru of the West, Marshall McLuhan, who reads and interprets our present. A group of "young" savants whose individual ages reach up into the eighties.

We might even bring in Mae West who, after twenty-seven years off the screen, came back in a controversial movie to upstage the screen's up-to-date sex goddess, Raquel Welch. And Mae was seventy-six when she did it.

So if we appear to be having a youth syndrome, it isn't youth itself that gives it meaning, but the quality of youth. The youth game is played with the rules that get you out of the syndrome. There are threads connecting it all, just as we are at a new awareness that there are cosmic threads linking us to the universe and all aspects of it. Instead of alienation, we are coming to accept that nothing is *un*related, and that everything exists in an interlocking chain.

Perhaps that is why in what follows you may find that there is really no one thought that ends by itself; it goes on to link with another.

Approaching a new century is always a challenge to man's imagination and the limitless reaches of his spirit. While we are asking the questions, the messages are coming in from all directions—known and unknown. One is unique in that it poses the question: Is it the beginning or the end?

Psychiatrists tell us that while pessimism is part of life, joy, too, is normal.

Right now, one of the outlooks for man is that he may not see the twenty-first century. On the contrary, there is the other possibility: that he will escape *into* the twenty-first century.

Kurt J. Wagner, M.D.
Beverly Hills, California

CONTENTS

*Observe always that everything
is the result of change, and
get used to thinking that there
is nothing Nature loves so well
as to change existing forms and
to make new ones like them.*

MARCUS AURELIUS

All About Modern
PLASTIC SURGERY
. . . and how you should feel about it
and YOURSELF

It is more than a result, it is both effect and affect. Winston Churchill used to say that we shape our buildings, and then they begin to shape us. Psychiatry and McLuhan have brought us to realize that the inside becomes what the outside reflects. The reflection in the mirror becomes the inner, as well as the outer, reality.

CHAPTER 1

Copemanship

A DOCTOR'S office is like a cross section of life. A plastic surgeon's office is more like a cross section of our time.

If this is the era of rearrangement of established truths, when Albert Einstein runs over Euclid by showing that parallel lines do meet, the youth-age lines do not create the neat geometric alienation we seem to have established for ourselves.

According to Marshall McLuhan and his colleagues in an article in *Harper's Bazaar*, April, 1968, entitled "Swinger vs. Square," the *Square* is frozen within the frame of a controlled environment. The *Swinger* is obedient to inner impulses, creating personal environments, expressing changing identities.

How can we know the dancer from the dance?

The young seem to have inherited the earth, not being meek about it, at that, but an earth child has been defined as a person who feels at one with today's struggle but has never resolved it in his own life.

One 25-year-old TV star who needed some facial reconstruction after an automobile accident was one of the most alienated human beings ever to come into my office. Causes he could get steamed up over, but there was nothing in his personal life he had ever found to relate to.

A woman of fifty said to me, "I have never felt so free in my life." She is not only part of her time, she is a living entity of its mainstream. This woman is what contemporaries half her age would call "together." She knows that the world around her belongs to her as much as to them, and she has an individual awareness of her relationship to it.

Myths we have lived with as gospel are being exploded—from "babies are not people, merely plastic blobs that take on the shape of society as they grow into it," to "sex is not a biological fact of life but some goody granted us at the approved time."

Exploding myths around her don't make this woman uncomfortable and anxiety-ridden. They liberate her. She is not losing a sense of values but is seeing them in the light of new ones. And she feels free because, instead of perceiving a mass of conflicts in a bewildering new kind of world, her mind is as open as her eyes.

In our viable language, this woman who is all in one piece might have been said, earlier in our cosmic revolution, to be with it. This denotes more a going along with what's happening, mindlessly or not, and wouldn't be accurate at all. *Together* is really more like it.

Perhaps the very progression from *with it* to *together* in itself indicates what's happening.

Age is really getting to be a relative thing. The present twenty-fives to thirty-fives who started the youth revolution are now earning their way *inside* the Establishment. The *under* twenty-fives to whom the world seemingly belongs are already on their way to joining them, whether they want to believe it or not.

The youth syndrome, by now, would seem to indicate that man is still inventing myths to live by. But it seems that in the lightning telescoping of time as we have come to know it, the myths seem to self-destruct before they can become part of the lore of reality.

14

It is the truth we come to, not the myth, that finally endures. Man is learning to be expansive, to reach for the possibilities. That's where the fountain of youth really fonts.

The fact is that while man's life span is increasing, the age span is leveling out, just as our class structures are leveling out.

Even the built-in rot of the view of life as being divided into thirds is coming in for revision. Schooling, work, decline into old age—what could be more rigid, more constricting, and more defeating to what man is really capable of?

Each man, every man. In the awareness of the flexibility of the individual, there will be no such sharp division. There will be no finishing of one phase and going on to the next, in which each step is designed to use *up* life, not to use it.

The flavor of egghead about the words, "You only go to school to learn *how* to learn (or to think)" was really only euphemistic. Education was actually considered to stop with the gaining of the diploma. Then on to the work that it prepared you for!

This locked-in life style was shaped to the idea that a man had so many work years in him, like a horse, and faced only retirement after that into an empty decline.

Sometime during the Industrial Revolution of the last century, when we changed from a rural civilization to an urban one, a different kind of work became the focal point of man's existence. He became necessary as a cog in the mechanized world we were making, as eventually women became necessary also. A man's work was supposed to be his life, and not to do an honest day's hard labor was a shameful thing.

This brings to mind the old man in a crowd surrounding the late Robert F. Kennedy, who said to him, "I understand you've never done a hard day's work in your life."

The Senator, understanding what the old man was getting at, grinned, "No, I guess I haven't."

"Son," said the old man, "don't let it bother you. You haven't missed a thing."

Our American civilization was built around the great nine-to-five day at the office or the factory. The six-day week became the five-day week, and now with many professional men taking Wednesdays off, the idea of the four-day week is becoming a general goal.

It was considered social progress, but it began to pose the question: What will we do with our leisure? Here man's life has been his job. Without it, he had so little within himself that to leave it was not liberation but a withering.

What it adds up to is that man, having been a slave to the necessities for survival, found that the emphasis had shifted to finding a *means* for survival.

In an age when he has progressed so far as to have engineered the means of his own destruction, man is prone to think he has reached the summit of civilization.

The fact is that he is only at the threshold of it. It has been illustrated that in point of time of the life of this planet, if the clock were set at 12 when man arrived (or evolved), it is now 12:15. In point of development, it is obvious that he is still a savage.

But the emphasis has shifted from a painful, slow evolution to a rocketing technology that has outstripped man's knowledge of himself. Is he to be the ruler, or the victim, like Frankenstein? Man, in some oversimplification, seems to have painted himself into a corner.

While the Establishment man tried to cope with unsolvable problems in the old ways and with the old methods, a new breed of native took over that said new ways have to be found. It is known not as the new generation, but the *now generation.*

Along with the rebellion, they even took on the look of a new breed of human. The peaked hats and oversized goggles that became a trademark were decidedly reminiscent of our former image of people from outer planets. And they seemed almost as strange and far removed from reality as we had known it.

This was the younger generation of the sixties. Each new generation expresses its rebellion against authority by creating its own freak fashions and fads and ideas. It is considered part of growing up, part of being oneself and not like father or mother.

But this one was different. Its relationship to the world it was born into was different. This generation seemed to have been born without the built-in respect for accepted social order. This wasn't rebellion, it was defiance. More, it was revolution. Or, evolution?

Ultimately, it became the first generation to turn down a war. This caused man to look at war—perhaps for the first time—and examine what he found in it. They, this new world force, believe they can make the kind of world they want if someone will listen.

It is easy to act without thinking. The individual's awareness of his own actions—and the possible result—is the meaningful element of change.

In this seemingly unthinking world, man is thinking furiously to get to know himself. And he is only on the verge—more like the sensing before a discovery—of knowing things about himself he had not even imagined previously.

More pertinent, science, heretofore considered nothing less than an exact entity, now finds that it is incomplete, groping, and it is beginning to realize its own mysticism.

We are finding immortality in the chemical elements that compose the universe—and discovering that each of us is a miniature universe. We are seeing things in new ways, and experiencing a mind expansion not brought on by drugs.

Life that has become an unbearable pressure cooker outside has forced man inside—to search for some semblance of peace within himself.

People, the people native to this new age, are learning to communicate by vibration. A philosophy not of reason but a philosophy of the East is moving in—one that deals with what man is inside himself in relation to his universal environment.

We are finding new worlds around us in which the supernatural becomes the natural. Figuratively, even literally, the old ghost story is taking on scientific substance. Mysticism and the occult and ESP—all parapsychological studies—are spreading. There are

17

situations we do not have answers for, but we are becoming solidly aware that they are there and people are experimenting.

We do know that electrical impulses, like the radio waves from outside the atmosphere, do emanate from humans. This is not only one more example of man's tie-in with his universe, but it gives us a basis for an explanation of extrasensory perception.

And science—not just people who like to free their imaginations—science, is saying that it is quite possible we may some day be communicating with each other by thought waves. Why not, when even now we sit in our houses and receive pictures transmitted through the air. It's called television.

If the new order seems to negate what we think in order to raise the importance of what we feel, it doesn't necessarily mean that we are sending 2,500 years of Aristotelian deductive reasoning down the drain.

It means, perhaps, that we are going on to discover new meanings even Ari didn't conjecture about, meanings that are deeper within man and his universe.

The new math is a sort of microcosmic math that equates everything not separately but as part of a universal whole.

Shakespeare sensed the power of this when he had Hamlet say, "There are more things in heaven and earth, Horatio, than are dreamt of in your philosophy."

Marshall McLuhan, the great guru who interprets our perplexing new age, takes it a more concrete step forward with his linear theory.

We are finding indications that there is, indeed, energy in form and line. There are strong indications that there is an answer to the age-old question, "Why were the pyramids built in their special shape?" There was a reason. It is said to be, and has been demonstrated in tests by scientists, because things ossify in that shape. So whatever died in those pyramids did not disintegrate, but ossified.

There is no question that man has gathered much knowledge that he has forgotten. Now he is rediscovering much of it based on

18

what would yesterday have been considered not science but séance material.

Man is also now facing such possibilities as being overwhelmed by the massive state and the massive corporation, or being annihilated either by his own neglect of his ecology or some hydrogen bomb. Whichever way he looks at it, he is likely to get it in the end.

But the universe is of such orderly, incredible magnitude that when man becomes disorderly, he must come back into order.

E. M. Forster, who examined the racial differences between the sensitive Indians and the Colonial Britons in his celebrated *A Passage to India*, seems to have preceded the current cult of investigating what the East has to give us. Some time before he died at 91, Forster said of the individual, "He seems to me a divine achievement and I mistrust any view which belittles him."

No matter how rotten man may claim man is, there is something about the spirit of man that remains indomitable.

We are at the fascinating point of either destroying ourselves—or moving into the golden era of existence in which man comes to understand himself.

Which is it to be? Like everything else that concerns the mystery of why man exists, nobody has the answer.

But who destroys man but himself? Until he learns to control his brain, which makes him act as he does, he has learned virtually nothing. But when he does, there can be a magnificence to man's fulfillment at which we cannot even begin to guess.

Life then will be not a struggle for survival but a shedding of the savage skin into a meaningful experience.

In the biggest cliff-hanger of all time, is man going to manage to survive to achieve it? Concern without optimism is nihilism. In the last third of this century we are hearing more and more statements beginning with "In the year 2,000. . . ."

Are we going to make it? I think it ought to be one hell of a New Year's Eve, the one that ushers it in.

19

CHAPTER 2

Happiness, Too, Is Inevitable

Albert Camus

MAN is an individual, not an age. He is capable of anything he believes he is capable of. He can be as relaxed and free as a Peter Max drawing, filled with design but reaching out to the bounds of infinity.

He can see the perfection and purity of a raindrop. There is an unrestrained happiness in it that seems to symbolize in its clarity what man has been looking for, what he can ultimately be.

The most intricate computer is the human brain. Nobody, except its original Creator, has ever built a computer that even begins to approximate the brain.

The brain is also a switchboard, plugged into by countless impressions constantly besieging the human organism, both from without and within. Emotions, for one, send their effects to every cell in the body.

The visio-audio sensory messages that the brain is constantly receiving do not get crumpled and thrown into the wastebasket after being read by the body. The body does not just say "I read you"; it sets up a chain reaction, like the ripples from a stone thrown in water.

Even our muscles register what we have in our psyches and they respond. That's why we walk free, or stiff, or funny; why we are graceful and effortless or clunky or jerky in our movements.

Life runs on electrical energy, and the brain is the converter of it. When we die, not all the organisms of the body die at once. Medicine accepts that we are dead when the brain is dead, when the electrical current is finally cut. Thus man lives within his brain. And it converts outer stimuli (from the environment) and inner stimuli (from the psyche) to make us what we are.

To take McLuhan's aphorism of our time, that the medium *is* the message, a step further: The mental image becomes the reality of the outer one.

It used to be the great truism that it was the inner qualities that counted and the outer ones were but superficial—as in the old saying that beauty is only skin deep. But we know now that there is no such thing as separating the mind from the body. The organism, like the Lord our God, is one.

When you look in the mirror and what you see doesn't match what you think you are—when the reflection is alienated from yourself—then the inner and outer selves are bound to have an effect on each other. The physical image becomes the mental reality.

Until now, we accepted as fact that the exterior was supposed to age—whether it matched the spirit in doing so or not. There was something disgraceful about not accepting the aging process "gracefully."

In their biological explorations, virtually all branches of medicine have come to the realization that aging is a disease that can be arrested. Today some of the best work in medicine is being directed to this end—not only to make life longer, but to make it better.

Cosmetic plastic surgery is today the visual equivalent of what medicine is working to accomplish inwardly. In the past decade, cosmetic operations have increased approximately 500 percent. Whether for improving the shape of a nose or getting the full face

22

lift treatment, over a half million persons have had beauty surgery during the last year.

The new approach to beauty surgery involves simply a pragmatic question-and-answer situation. Not "Why do I want it," as in the past, but "What can I do and how do I get it?"

While this progress has led into pragmatism, I hope the deeper, more emotional intangible is not lost with it.

Something happens with plastic surgery that is not only cosmetic; it brings a new element into existence. I have yet to perform a face lift that did not also lift the patient into a new awareness of life.

Our electronic age, as with everything else, has given us a lively awareness of beauty surgery. There used to be something esoteric and unreachable about what those figures on the silver screen did to keep looking that way. But those figures coming into your living room on TV achieve a three-dimensional familiarity, like real, *human* people.

Have you, too, been going out of your skull over those newly blooming, fresh-as-a-rose faces all over your television screen?

All of a sudden, overnight, there she is—the panel show regular, the actress, the singer—the familiar female of whom you can say that over a span of maybe fifteen years "I've grown accustomed to her face"—sporting a new one as dewy as the rose freshly bloomed. What's more, it looks right into the camera, lingering under the exploratory closeup with the smooth serenity of a pussycat.

Whereas before, if you were tuned in to such stuff, you could pick out *a* face that had had "something" done, now it's virtually everybody. Endemic, newly minted youth has become a mind bender.

But in our world of participation and involvement, what a woman sees on the screen she knows she can get for herself. And she has an investment in making the most of herself to make the most of her life. The youth-oriented "secrets" of the specialized have become an open sesame for suburbia.

23

Case histories have moved on from the aging actress whose career was saved by her plastic surgeon to the career woman who was going to lose *her* job if she didn't stop falling apart in the face to the housewife who is becoming a disaster area and doesn't want to lose her husband.

In our classless society, the access is no longer restricted to those with money and leisure, nor to the worlds of entertainment and the beautiful people.

In Europe, beauty surgery is looked upon openly and honestly for what it is: something available to the human being to make life better.

In Brazil it is a status symbol to have your face lifted. And when you go all the way and have beauty surgery on your body—such as the "riding breeches" operation to remove the fat flaps on your thighs or a stomach lift—you're really *in.*

When letters come in with problems that can only be answered by plastic surgery, I know that I made the only decision possible for me when I decided at the age of nine that was I going to be a plastic surgeon.

I seem to have been predestined for it in two ways. To begin with, I am the fifth generation of doctors straight down from my great-great-grandfather, who went back to the days when doctors were really barber-surgeons. This great-great was, in fact, one of the few practicing surgeons in the early nineteenth-century history of Viennese medicine.

My great-grandfather was a general practitioner. His son, my grandfather, became an obstetrician as well as a notorious abortionist, a practice not looked on with delight in Catholic Vienna.

My father is, of course—by this time in Viennese medical history, what else?—a practicing psychiatrist.

If I seem to be a product of this history of Viennese medicine—from barber-surgeons to psychiatry—it is not undiluted with still earlier diplomacy.

Another of my great-greats is still hanging around Vienna's Schonnbrun Palace, or his bust is, anyway. He is listed in the

Encyclopaedia Britannica in various versions of his full name, Kaunitz-Rietberg, Wenzel Anton, Prince von, Prince Chancellor to Maria Theresa, 1711-94.

It is the latter fact that has made family history over political history, because the old boy is considered to have been more than just chancellor to Maria Theresa, despite the fact that she herself is cited for her exemplary family life and her sixteen children, one of whom was Marie Antoinette.

During his chancellorship he managed such things as the Austrian-French coalition against Frederick the Great in the Seven Years' War and the alliance between Austria and France during his ambassadorship to France (1750-52).

Oh, it was Kaunitz' own granddaughter who married Metternich in 1795, thereby bringing to full circle the fact that it was Kaunitz who had carried the first outline of the young Metternich in the first dispatch to Maria Theresa. If you want to piece this part of European-Austrian history together, look them up: Metternich, Maria Theresa, Kaunitz. It's even more fascinating now that you know about Wenzel and Maria!

The union of Germany and Austria *(Anschluss)* occurred on March 11, 1938—two days after my fourth birthday. Whereupon my family did what they had been contemplating since 1934— they got the hell out and came to this country.

It would have happened sooner, under which circumstances I would have been born in the U.S., and not Austria. But there was some sort of a complicated family involvement with money coming to my mother, and she didn't want to leave without it.

As it turned out, it didn't make any difference. The Nazis confiscated the money anyway. My father had $75 in his pocket when we found our new *pied à terre* on Kosciusko Street.

From all of this, I wound up on Kosciusko Street in Booklyn's Bedford-Stuyvesant area—which makes up for its lack of any aristocratic pretense with toughness. In this melting pot you had to hold your own or else.

The Italians beat me up because I wasn't Italian, the blacks

25

because I was white, the Irish because they thought I was a Jew, and the Jews because they thought I was a Nazi.

It was here, at age nine, that I discovered what *kind* of doctor I was to be. I had been sent down to the corner candy store for the evening newspaper. Among the paperback books on the racks was one by Maxwell Maltz. Yes, even then, pre-Psychocybernetics, he was the writing plastic surgeon, inspiring people to look inwardly to find themselves. I am not even certain about the title, any more, but something in that book got to my nine-year-old mind.

I was so carried away by this new world I had uncovered that by the time I got home—in spite of all the dither about where I had been so long—my whole future was settled. Even this book may be a direct result of the example set by Maxwell Maltz.

My father did not, as it would be nice to say, go into psychiatric practice right away in New York, but he did find a full-time job with Uncle Sam for the duration of World War II.

My mother—well, my mother is really something special, being a woman. I learned compassion for women from my mother—for the way they think and for their special needs.

She talked to me about the difference between men and women. I don't mean the difference in *vive la différence.* There is a lot of difference between men and women aside from anatomy.

They are biologically different and, therefore, emotionally and mentally so. The trouble comes when one sex expects the other to act in his or her way when they aren't constituted that way at all. This is what accounts for a lot of the puzzlement and frustration between the sexes, and what some people never let themselves understand.

My mother understands this, and she thought it was important that I did, about the difference between men and women. As a consequence, I think I am peculiarly constituted emotionally to empathize with a woman who comes to me as a patient and says, "I am not a woman because I haven't any breasts."

As another footnote to the past that I still carry with me, there are the religions in my background.

My mother, who is Catholic, and being a woman, is more perspicacious than my Jewish father, compromised about not leaving Austria in 1934. With Hitler's hot breath blowing from Germany, she decided to take a chance and wait it out for the money, though she took no chance on me—I was baptized a Catholic.

You want to know about religion? I have kept on learning about it all my life. Sometimes being on both sides of the religious coin can be rather bewildering but helpful.

It's tough enough for a plastic surgeon to find a residency at any time. When I was in Oklahoma City trying to make my own residency, I almost lost it because I was *Jewish,* until I made it a point to mention to the chief of surgery that I knew the bishop.

Later in New York I got my residency because I *was* Jewish, and I never mentioned the bishop.

Actually, I consider that I served my real residency while a captain at Wright-Patterson Air Force Base, Dayton, Ohio, as chief of plastic surgery there from 1964 to 1966.

It would be hard, if not impossible, to match in private practice the spectrum of surgery I did for those Air Force men and their families.

It ranged from congenital anomalies in infants to repair of the 62-year-old mother of an Air Force sergeant who had set fire to herself smoking a cigarette and was brought in with third degree burns on fifteen percent of her body, including the upper torso and arms.

This vital, successful reconstructive surgery became part of my written submission of case histories when I was standing for certification by the American Board of Plastic Surgeons. Just recently I was called in on emergency for a case of burns where the patient was at the point of death. It was almost identical to that of the Air Force sergeant's 62-year-old mother. This woman recovered and I gave *her* a face lift, too.

It was in July, 1966, having served my tour of duty with the Air Force, that I opened my office in Beverly Hills.

27

Anyone starting out in a professional field today, especially if it is an established one—and there is *no* field more established than medicine—comes up against conditions he would like to change. While other professions may realize that progress is won by experimentation, medicine carries with it the conditioning to stick to what has been proved and *not* to experiment, not in practice, anyway.

By virtue of what medicine deals with—human life—progress through experiment becomes a sticky wicket. But in a world getting so thoroughly unstuffed in all directions, even the traditionally conservative world of medicine must yield to the new needs of a changing era of man. Things possible can no longer be ignored, or made to wait. Life itself is moving too fast to wait, as tomorrow becomes today.

If I have been known as a rebel at times in my own comparatively short tenure in the medical establishment, I have been a rebel working for change *within* the Establishment.

This is truly the age of protest, when it is possible not to believe that the American Medical Association is the gospel according to Hippocrates.

We have, after all, possibly the first older generation ever to be influenced by the younger. Hopefully, it may even happen in medicine.

However, it is also part of the nature of man to distrust and fear change because he doesn't understand it. This makes it a *confused* world. And woman, never too sure of the world or her status in it since the beginning of time, is perhaps the most confused, although men have their bewilderments too.

Probably no one is more in a position to be aware of this than a plastic surgeon.

Nothing is more confusing to the psyche than the progressive appearances of aging itself—when a woman or man looks in the mirror and a seeming stranger looks back.

Something is there that wasn't there before. The first shock comes, perhaps, toward the late thirties: there are the new

28

wrinkles around the lower eyelids and the beginning crow's feet at the outer corners of the eyes.

In the very late thirties and the forties there is the progression to neck wrinkling and the deepening of the nasolabial folds stretching from nose to mouth spelling age.

Toward the late forties the deepening has changed to a new look altogether. The tender contours of the face have changed to deep set dewlaps—appealing on a basset hound, horrific on the human.

And then it's all happened—the frown lines, the forehead "car tracks," the bags under the eyes and the sagging mouth that seems to feel their weight, the pouches breaking up the formerly clean, smooth chin line, the jowls that go with the dewlaps, the double chin or neck stringiness (depending on whether you are fat or thin), the ear lobes that elongate, and the widening of a swan neck into a wrestler's.

Atrophic skin changes are working in conjunction with these newly established gravitational and dynamic lines. The skin becomes that characteristic dull, yellowish tan, the pigmentation spotty, the skin tone scaly, dry and inelastic.

Now, for the first time, you realize the heart-touching anguish of seeing one of nature's prime delights—the dewy, magnificent rose, yesterday just budding, today a withered droop of petals on the stalk. And you ponder it, perhaps for the first time.

Yet, does anyone like to speak of a shriveled rose? Of course not. Even the Last Rose of Summer was left blooming!

The image you carry of yourself should never shrivel either. The process of living itself leaves an imprint on the personality that is imposed on all aspects of the person. That is perhaps what living *can* become: a personality development, not a deterioration of the inner and outer person.

It is considered—and really is—foolish for a woman of sixty to want to look twenty. Even if she could, it would not match her *being,* her development as a person—and why should she want to negate that?

29

To look a *fit* sixty is a pleasure for the world, and it does wonders for the mental image of the one who has reached that age. The beautiful part of beauty surgery, when it is accomplished properly, is that there is no startling transformation. It is simply a removal of deterioration, so that those around you do not say, "You look so *different*," but can say with pleasure, "You look so well."

There is no confusion where there is awareness of self and the relationship of that self to the environment. The real "secret" of agelessness is in the discovery of self. And the ageless person is becoming the new fact of life.

As a matter of fact, youth is wonderful, beauty is a blessing, but in the end, agelessness is better than both.

It says that happiness, too, is inevitable.

CHAPTER 3

Who Is a Plastic Surgeon?

THERE is in my office a sculpture of one Tagliocozzi, who is doing a nose graft from the skin of the forearm, circa 1576.

Today, with plastic surgery one of the most proliferating branches of medicine, it isn't really that people don't know, but they still want to be told the answer so they can be sure they *do* know: What is the difference between a plastic surgeon, a beauty surgeon, and a cosmetic surgeon?

Good old Taglio, extending that piece of skin, like a string, from the forearm to the nose back there in 1576 exemplifies the answer.

They are all the same. A plastic surgeon does reconstructive work on the human anatomy that also beautifies. Much reconstructive work is not done for the purpose of beautifying, but anything that is made whole and right and functional again is beautified in the process. In the same sense, beauty surgery is reconstructive surgery as well. Hence it can be said that a plastic surgeon uses his skills and knowledge to specialize in beauty surgery. It is an interlocking chain.

31

All medical terms for plastic surgery are from the Greek, beginning with *plastis* itself, meaning to sculpt or mold. Yet so literal-minded is the layman that one woman, going home from the hospital still bandaged from such surgery, was asked by the cab driver, "When does the plastic come off?"

The cabbie wasn't so far off, at that. In the constant search for new materials and better techniques among the bone and cartilage banks of natural materials and man-made materials as well, plastics are found to be more and more satisfactory to implant in man. Not, of course, to "come off," but for permanency.

While there are certain conditioned ethics *within* plastic surgery, there are no firmly established guide lines as to just who *is* a plastic surgeon. Perhaps that accounts for the confusion and uncertainty in the mind of the patient seeking a plastic surgeon.

For instance, *any* regular, run-of-the-mill M.D. can legally perform plastic surgery. But a plastic surgeon is a surgical specialist. After his four years of medical school and one year of internship, the aspiring plastic surgeon has three years of general surgical training, followed by at least another two years of training in plastic surgery. Once he has had two years of practice in plastic surgery, he is eligible to take the examinations to be certified by the American Board of Plastic Surgery.

Of the approximately 10,000 plastic surgeons now practicing in the U.S., there are about 1,200 certified by the American Board. I was number 674—and I was certified in 1966, five years before this was written—so it is obvious that the mills of the gods do grind slowly in accepting qualified new plastic surgeons.

Less than ten percent of practicing plastic surgeons are certified by the American Board of Plastic Surgery, and there is even some confusion about who is certified by which board, since each branch of specializing medicine (including plastic surgery) has its own board. There is in addition to the American Society of Plastic and Reconstructive Surgeons (of which a separate board passes on eligibility of members), the American Society of Facial Plastic Surgeons, who deal only with facial surgery.

An eye-ear-nose-and-throat man, about to do a rhinoplasty, for

32

example, can answer, "Yes" when asked if he is certified by *the* Board.

There is even a case on record of one plastic surgeon, a former osteopath, who formed his own board, published a periodical, and made himself president, with his own office as the address.

A *qualified* plastic surgeon is as qualified to remove a gall bladder as he is to rebuild a face. If he did, the chances are you would come out of it with a more aesthetic suturing!

The plastic surgeon's sensitive, highly developed fingers are adapted to dealing with reconstructions ranging from paralysis of facial nerves to abdominal wall defects to the ravages of burns.

As a captain at Wright-Patterson Air Force Base hospital, where I had a great deal of "experience" as chief of plastic surgery, there were these and many, many others that had to be dealt with. Congenital anomalies, from correcting the cleft lip and palate of a 2½-month-old infant, to a bilateral syndactylism (joining of the ring and long fingers) of a 22-month-old boy, to adult male hypospadias were among my cases.

To simplify, the last-named is a congenital condition in which the urethra does not extend far enough into the penal shaft, affecting sexual as well as biological functioning. Depending on the individual case, this can involve anything from skin grafts, to building up the tube, to more flap at the end of the penis.

Although not usually congenital, the opposite of this would be one of the major troubles that beset the female vagina. And it is more horrifying than amazing to realize how little is known, in our own otherwise knowledgeable society, about how much can be done for such conditions. Actually, almost everything can be done. That's why I was more happy than amused at Mario Puzo's description in *The Godfather* of a *perincorrhaphy*—the repairing of the pelvic sling.

What author Puzo had to say about the connection between this form of virtual sexual castration for a female and suicide, has a frustrating validity. Even though it may not end in suicide, the mental and physical anguish must be inestimable—and quite needless.

33

The atonic vagina or monstrously oversized vagina, as Puzo had it for literary reasons—can be tightened even when there is no sphincter action, by repairing the top and bottom walls. There are even skin graft vaginas substituted for damaged ones that come to work normally. A mushy vagina *can* be made into a more muscular, younger organ.

This simple knowledge could change the miserable lives of countless women who just take it for granted that nothing can be done. There seems to be an inbuilt feeling of guilt or shame about the genitalia that keeps a patient from asking even her doctor's advice.

For the first such operation I performed I insisted that the woman's own gynecologist be present. She had not asked him about it but broached the subject to me while consulting me about her face.

Today's great liberation is reaching into these heretofore guilt-ridden areas, too. The very newest field in plastic surgery is, in fact, sexual surgery. From building vaginas from virtually nothing there is the opposite number—"member" is perhaps the better word—of a permanent surgical cure for impotence.

Before you smell the snake oil in such a statement, let me say that it can be done, although it isn't all as miraculous as it sounds in saying so. The simple explanation of how it's done is by inserting a silicone strut into the penis, so that there is a permanent sort-of erection; sort-of, but still workable. One man who came to me to be made potent again asked, "But, doctor, if it's there all the time, how do I walk?" I replied, "Not too well."

The truth is, this is one operation that should be looked on as a last, not a first resort. When you're fooling around with putting foreign bodies in the penis for no pathologic necessity, both doctor and patient should be very sure not so much of *what* they're doing, but *why.*

Aside from the potency factor, I have had patients complain that the penis is too small (never too big!), so could I make it larger? The fact is, a very large member can be quite painful to the

34

sex partner. There is that mythful pride in size, when actually, the truth of the situation is not the size at all; I tell these prospective patients that it is not the horse alone, but the jockey as well, who wins the race.

The fact is that sex is so tied up with the psyche that ninety-eight out of 100 such cases are invalid. Potency is not a silicone strut but the man himself. The same man who cannot achieve an erection with his wife of twenty-seven years may have no trouble at all with a tempting, young body. The sexual hangup is not in the sex organ.

Such hangups may run from temporary to deep-seated, requiring intensive psychotherapy. Any man who has come to me to change his sex organ in some way needs *some* kind of psychiatric help. There was the man who came in looking like a banker, who turned out to need quite a bit. He wanted a larger penis. As he talked, his whole demeanor changed. "I want to let my hair down," he told me, "I'll let it all hang out." I didn't have to be a practicing psychiatrist to know immediately that what this man needed was a couch, not an operating table.

Nonetheless, the fact that these operations are possible enlarges the field of plastic surgery to still further horizons. The most dramatic is still, of course, the transsexual operation, the man being made physically into a woman. The piquant question here is does he only pass for a woman? Or is *she* really a woman?

I have performed only one transsexual operation myself. It was an operation I do not want to do again. The first thing I did was cut off his penis. I could hardly bring myself to do it. Regardless of the surgical training, there is something about this particular surgery that goes beyond training and conditioning.

How I came to do this particular operation was that he was a patient of mine who kept at me to do the operation that would make him a woman, which to himself he was psychically already.

I kept telling him to go to Denmark, and he kept insisting. Surgically, I knew I could handle it. I had amputated cancerous scrotums (not the same as amputating the penis!), and there had been hypospadias and atonic vaginas. I had a pretty thorough working knowledge of the genitalia and their biological connections, so I couldn't see why this operation actually would differ so drastically from some of the others that can be done. Since I expect this to be my first and last transsexual case, and since I have already gone into it this far, I might go on to explain that from the scrotum I made him a vagina; and even a clitoris fashioned from the gland of the penis.

The result was—I am giving you the answer!—operative and functional. As to what degree it was sexually workable, that was, of course, up to the patient and her new sex partner.

The amount of intensive psychotherapy and other therapy involved in the transsexual operation is too much for a general plastic surgeon to undertake. If any man really wants to go through with all the complications of becoming a woman (no woman has yet attempted becoming physically a man that I have heard of), I advise him that this is a very special type of operation indeed, and that he should be in one of the university hospitals doing special research on the subject.

There is one respect in which the plastic surgeon is unique. He is a "happy doctor." The only other kind of doctor who can be included in this category is the obstetrician. Both bring happiness with something that is *wanted*—something you can see and feel and touch and enjoy on a daily basis.

A plastic surgeon has a great opportunity for a personal relationship with his patients, possibly more than a doctor does in any other medical field. What he accomplishes is not something mysteriously clinical—the details of which the patient will never actually be quite sure of—but something tangible that can be seen, discussed, admired, and enjoyed as part of a heightened awareness of life.

Yet the grand old men of plastic surgery, instead of realizing this joy unique to their own specialty, too often have maintained the traditional aloof mystique acquired with the taking of the Hippocratic oath. This, too, is changing however. The doctor or surgeon is no longer a remote entity on a pedestal, practically deified. He is becoming more of a skilled technician, dealing with human values as well as human bodies.

With a more informed and aware public, patients are meeting their doctors on a more human-to-human rather than human-to-God basis. The results should be a freer give-and-take that will help to bridge the gap between layman and professional.

Who knows? Doctors may even overcome that unconscious hostility factor almost built in with most patients. The hostility is, of course, the result of having to get medical help in the first place. It means there is something wrong—a mystery and therefore something to be afraid of—which you cannot cope with alone, and which you would much rather do without.

But plastic surgery is something you *do* want in the first place, which is why you are in the surgeon's office, apprehensive, but with a surging spirit of hope and optimism that is far stronger than the apprehension.

Another unique aspect of plastic surgery is that although ostensibly it deals with aging, its whole outlook is toward youth. Although this doesn't make it mandatory that the surgeon be young, it helps if the surgeon *thinks* young. There is no other branch of medicine in which thinking "young" is so much a part of the whole ambience for both doctor and patient—and which has such an effect on the total result.

Yet, so far there is little evidence in the ethos of plastic surgery of this orientation of matching the psychology to the treatment. In the practice of medicine, if you had to pick a one-word rule, it would be: conform. Conform to the tried, the tested and (supposedly) the true. Or, if you're going to err, err on the side of safety. By the very nature of practicing medicine, caution is mandatory. But caution can be so ingrained as to mean immobility.

Time changes everything eventually, *even* in medicine—else there would be no progress. And in this era when change is so rapid as to create a revolution, even the sacrosanct practice of medicine must adjust its time clock.

Progress medically has always been hard won. The witch burning with each step forward is historically notorious. As one case in point, witness the trouble Louis Pasteur had with the august French Academy.

In my own field, the lay public is moving far ahead of the profession. The great paucity of plastic surgeons in relation to the demand will in itself have to bring revisions.

This is not to say that the Generation Gap is everywhere, even in medicine, but only that some air has to be let into what has grown to be a venerably stuffy Establishment.

Last year, about a half million people underwent cosmetic surgery of some kind. With the new awareness and shedding of old mental blocks, the number is growing astronomically. Yet this fastest growing area of medicine is developing no more than 130 new plastic surgeons a year—at a time when there are not nearly enough old ones to take care of the present demand itself.

Again, there are only loose guide lines for training new doctors—it is far too difficult for those who are newcomers. The new man, after three years of general surgery, gets those adamantly required two years of extra training in plastic surgery the best way he can.

He may be on a hospital staff, or he may be taken into the office where some established plastic surgeon is his preceptor, just as a young lawyer often works in the office of a judge.

Even after he has surmounted those two hard years of specialized training and goes into the two years of practice necessary before he can be certified, he may find it difficult to get on the staff of a hospital where he can operate. I had my own uphill struggle, but in the matter of being on a hospital staff, I guess I was one of the lucky ones.

One of the established conventions is, in fact, the matter of the hospital. A plastic surgeon who operated in his surgery in his own office has in the past been suspect; the aura was of something not quite ethical. He couldn't be on the staff of a hospital if he operated in his office; therefore he couldn't be "approved" by the best standards. In fact, one of the ways that the Old School made it tough for developing new plastic surgeons was by withholding hospital privileges.

By now, the status of the hospital itself is changing so drastically as to make this still accepted requirement for the hospital ridiculous. To begin with, aside from the overcrowded conditions, the cost of the operating room alone now runs $100 an hour, and costs are going up.

Say whatever you're in for takes an average of three to 3½ hours. (Somehow, it always seems to take longer in the hospital than in the office surgery.) Add to that basic the cost of the hospital room—anywhere from two to ten days, depending on the surgeon's *modus operandi*—and the ancillary services of the hospital and doctor, and nurses, if necessary.

Even if the heavy financial cost is not a factor, however, there are many general reasons why the old unwritten law of the hospital stay needs rewriting. First, there is the unnecessary danger, even likelihood, of being exposed to infection needlessly. Where hospital surgery is absolutely necessary, then, of course, you go to the hospital—and hope for the best.

But plastic surgery is a specialized surgery that you *elect* to have of your own free, yearning will—with hope in your soul and a soar in your spirit. Even to be in the next bed to a patient seriously and unpleasantly ill—or subjected to all the other sick-oriented codicils of a hospital stay—is simply not in keeping with the premise of having yourself made lovelier to look at.

Il faut souffrir pour être belle is an everlasting truism of the ages—we do, and we *will,* suffer to be beautiful—but it is a hopefully self-imposed temporary suffering we bear happily for the result, a different kind of suffering entirely from that which is associated with hospitals.

Because of overcrowded, overcostly, and often difficult conditions, a trip to the hospital should be reserved only for necessary health surgery such as a *cholecystectomy* and its ilk. A gall bladder removal is a different matter again from usual plastic surgery.

I give my patients an option; ninety percent elect to have the operative work done in my surgery, right in the familiar office, under a local anesthetic.

If a general anesthetic is required, then the hospital *is* the only alternative. Hospitals are necessary. I am not against them, but only to having the patient exposed to the prevailing conditions—unless unavoidable.

Further, a local anesthetic entails less risk of bleeding and subsequent infection, reduces bronchial complications, and allows for a more "natural" appearance following surgery. Post-operative misery and distress are considerably less than with a general anesthetic, making the patient's return to normal activity easier or the stay in the hospital shorter.

I not only *prefer* to operate in my own surgery under a local anesthetic, I am a therapeutic nihilist. I do not believe in medicine just for the sake of prescribing medicine. We excrete so many superfluous vitamins as it is, that we can only absorb so much of the super amounts taken. Our sewerage is often loaded with it. And that is not to say that it's healthy sewerage.

But I am not a Spartan either. As a matter of fact, I believe that any unnecessary pain attendant to plastic surgery is not good for the end result. Just as a pregnancy should be spiritually happy and healthy, plastic surgery recovery should have that same soaring outlook toward the future that might occur at other times in our lives: at graduation, getting married, and—sometimes—anniversaries! Some discomfort, perhaps, is necessary, but not pain.

There is generally so little pain that patients commonly refer to the medication that is given as a "forgetfulness" pill. What it is, of course, is a twilight sleep (drug induced), under which the patient may be aware of, but not bothered by, what is going on.

Afterwards, you have medication to keep any pain under control and to get lots of sleep. And you can do that much more comfortably at home than in a hospital.

So when you consult a plastic surgeon, don't ask him whether he performs his surgery in his office or in a hospital. At least, not until you've looked at his credentials. They are your first guide lines; the man himself, and the rapport you feel between you, the second. The old established values are something to live by, but they must be readjusted to what is realistic now. Like some outmoded social values, even established medical values can become anachronistic in themselves before the preceptors realize it.

The very insistence on existing mores, and that they be unchanging—thereby maintaining a set standard—is what makes it possible, oddly enough, for so many sub-standard plastic surgery mishaps which I see almost every working day. With the permissiveness—and strangely enough, that is the word for it—on the one hand, that *any* M.D. can perform plastic surgery, and on the other, the rigidity about accepting qualified young *surgeons,* the wonder is that the young men elect the hardships and the years of specialized training.

Under the *status quo,* the old men can do no wrong and the young men can do no right. To set high standards is necessary, but it is time to take some of the *quo* out of the *status.* If that be insurrection, make the most of it.

Even the most reactionary are slowly coming around to the order of things as they should be, not as they have wanted them to be.

The only answer is to let qualified men practice plastic surgery so as to ease the shortage that allows *un*qualified men to do the damage that must be answered for. It's still a good part of the conditioning to make a young man prove himself by making it tough for him. But it ought not to be impossible.

A greater autonomy will make it possible for plastic surgery to add joyous possibilities to life as a matter of course.

The shape of the future is looming up. From the old, adamant requirement of general hospital residency, more and more established surgeons are dreaming of setting up their own clinics. The day will certainly come when the *thing* will be not to have your plastic surgery done in a hospital at all, but in a private clinic.

The rich participate in the *now* of things as they will be tomorrow, and those who could afford it have been going to those little hideaway clinics in Europe for years as a matter of course.

41

The doctor's own surgery is today's forerunner of that. The clinic entirely devoted to maintaining the human physiology will be the actuality of tomorrow.

One of the reasons many of the privileged used to have their plastic surgery done in Europe was that there was less chance of running into people one knew at the wrong time or place—and giving away the "secret."

With today's acceptance of the whole procedure as a fact of life, however, the plastic surgeon's office has a casual, matter-of-fact atmosphere where a secretary and an actress can be waiting *vis-à-vis* for their appointments. The door they leave by, leading out of my office, is a convenience—not a cover-up.

When *Look* magazine interviewed me for an article on plastic surgery for men, the writer asked me if I thought plastic surgeons looked better, as a breed, than other men.

I said yes, they did. Would you want a plastic surgeon with a pouchy jawline to operate on you?

No, it's not done with mirrors. A plastic surgeon has another plastic surgeon operate on him, just as anyone else does. In my own case, I have had hair implants to cover what I have already lost, too early, alas, and a chin augmentation.

About the chin. I had grown a beard of which I was very fond. But I am a real eclectic about the new clothes freedom (I have been known to show up for an emergency call in the liberated clothes I had been wearing, thereby causing the already worried family some undue alarm at first meeting). My wife thought that the clothes were okay, but she insisted that the beard should go. I told a colleague, "I'll get rid of the beard if you give me that chin augmentation I think I need." The deal was too good for him to pass up.

Not only the plastic surgeon makes the most of things as they are but his family does as well. I did a blepharoplasty and a face lift for my mother at the same time. Then I did my father's eyes to match up with mother's.

My brother has had hair transplants, his nose fixed, and his chin pushed *back*. In his case, the chin was the opposite of mine.

Instead of needing a bit of augmentation, he had the prognathic jaw that called for a resectioning and a retraction of the chin.

As for my wife, she was already so attractive that when I met her I was prompted to say, "You're a very pretty girl, but you have *blepharorochlasis.*" She looked around to see what it was, as if her clothes had become disarranged or something anti-social like that.

Kathie was one of those people born with bags under the eyes. Pretty as she was—and perhaps layman's eyes wouldn't spot the necessity for it—my aesthetic sense wanted to pin her ears back and give her a bit more chin. Strangely enough, none of those things had bothered her at all. Eventually, I did them all, along with a mammaplasty—because she wanted *it.*

I made a deal. I exchanged the breast augmentation she wanted for the eyes, ears, and chin that I wanted. They were done at one sitting, in about 2½ hours.

Kathie is now so plastic-surgery mad that she can't wait to have something else done—only she can't figure out *what.* She keeps saying, "I am going to have a face peel next."

And she will, even if not for some time yet.

You see, Kathie has discovered the truth of the ages: that great beauties are made, not born.

CHAPTER 4

The Profile Analysis

Q. E. D. Anything in Harmony Is Pleasing

AESTHETIC surgery is a geometric study of proportions. Keats'
poetic insight that "beauty is truth, truth beauty" was matched
geometrically by the sculptor Schadow. In the nineteenth century
he formulated the facial proportions for a prevailing standard of
symmetry which the occidental world accepts as the ideal.

Our own eyes automatically accept the standard of what is
aesthetically pleasing. Take any super example—from Greta Garbo
to Rock Hudson—to even *any* example of the good-looking individual, and you know they pass the Schadow test before you
apply the calipers.

The sculptor formulated the measurements for perfection in
sculpture. But plastic surgery is sculpture for the living, the
Galatea legend given truth. So what has come to be accepted as
the Schadow canon becomes the "profile analysis" of the plastic
surgeon.

As any art student today knows, the Schadow canon divides the
face horizontally from eyebrows to chin in six equal parts, the

45

nose occupying three of these, the upper lip one, and the lower lip and chin two (see Figure 1).

Schadow Standard of Proportion

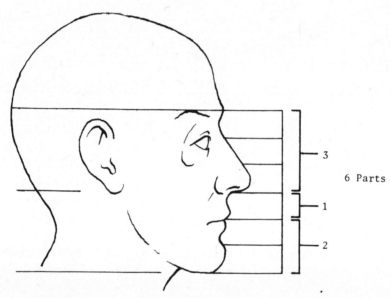

6 Parts

FIGURE 1. *The face, from eyebrow to lower border of chin, is divided into six equal parts, of which the nose occupies three, the upper lip one and the chin two. For a successful plastic surgery result, the proper proportions should be achieved.*

The perfect contour shows its truth by hitting a perpendicular line (which you can test yourself very simply, by laying a flat line, such as a ruler, along the root of the nose).

In Figure 2, under the Schadow, or perhaps in the Schadow standard of proportion, is shown a profile that does not lay claim at all to these standards, and the pencil markings that bring it up to par. The nose now takes off at the standard 30-35 degree angle, and the naso-labial angle at 90.

The Profile Analysis

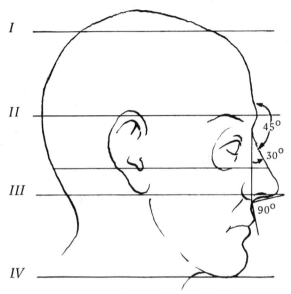

FIGURE 2. Horizontal lines, I to IV divide the face into its ideal proportions. The angles are measured with the head in horizontal position; variations of a few degrees are acceptable. Nose—lip angle should be 90°—95°. Forehead-nose angle should be 30°—35°.

The profile analysis indicates the necessity for a definite proportion between the forehead, nose, lips, and chin. To correct a nose alone, without considering the related features, is going on a fool's journey.

Sometimes it *is* the nose alone that needs correcting. Sometimes it can seem that the nose is out of line when it is really not the nose, but the chin—receding from or exceeding the profile analysis ideal.

Sometimes—a great deal of the time—it is *both* that need to be brought into harmony with the total face.

And if you examine successful before-and-after pictures, it is

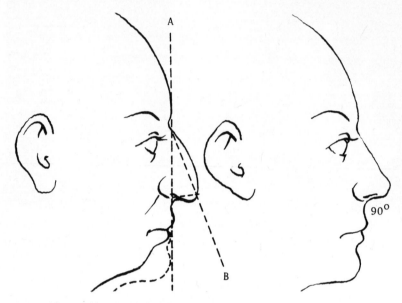

FIGURE 3.   *Profile before nose correction and with plumb line from nose root showing how it is brought into line with Schadow standard. The profile angle of 30 degrees is based on dotted line, A, and bridge line, B. When chin is recessed, as on the "before" drawing, the angle is increased, emphasizing the nose. The normal proportion is achieved by augmentation of the chin by 15 degrees.*

obvious that a former so-so lip line is brought into a more pleasing naso-labial angle with the correction of either nose or chin.

Does this sculpturized concept of beauty create a cold uniformity with the impersonal quality of sculpture itself? In the first place, there *is* nothing remote about a fine piece of sculpture— therefore so much for that conditioned bit of fallacy. A sculpture always bears the imprint of the artist, the inanimate materials of his art taking on a live malleability.

In the living sculpture of plastic surgery, it is the personality and original composition of the human that makes the difference;

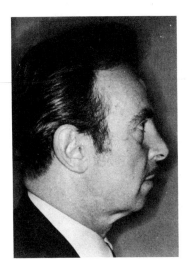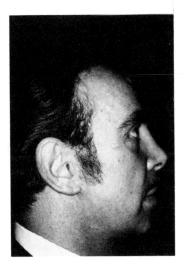

47-year-old man who had face lift, rhinoplasty, eye-lid lift, as well as chin augmentation. Result at six months.

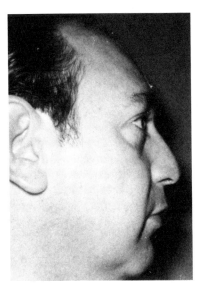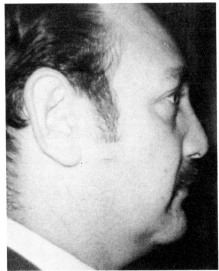

38-year-old male after chin enlargement with a slight modification of his nose. Result at six months.

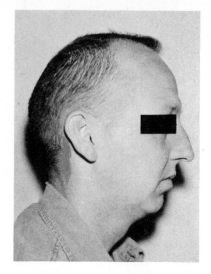 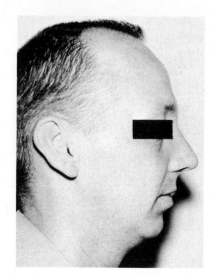

35-year-old male who had a rhinoplasty but would not have a chin
enlargement. Imagine the result if a
chin enlargement had been done.

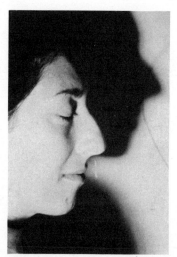 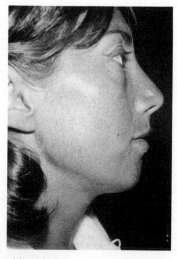

33-year-old female with a rhinoplasty. Result good, but look what a
chin operation could have accomplished.

it is retained within the framework of the ideal. No two works of art were ever alike, just as one of the prime factors of life is that no human being duplicates another.

A "bad" plastic surgery result can simply mean that the surgeon has not taken the greatest and basic quality—the individual conformation—into reckoning.

Sometimes the individual quality is so strong as to make a unique perfection of its very own. This is true in the case of "appealingly ugly" men. Men, in our social criteria, do not really need to be handsome. Yet if you apply critical standards to one of these rugged individualists, you may find that he will still fall into the Schadow canon of "truth" in formation. It is just his own personal, rugged overlay that gives it a different aspect.

And just as it is the exception that proves the rule, sometimes it is the imperfection that makes the attractiveness.

There are two prime examples of females who would never make the profile analysis ideal. And who never should! They are the non-conformists who are true originals. To tamper with their unique brand of special appeal would be to destroy a one-of-a-kind piece of artistry.

Of course, *the* name that has become a trademark for non-conforming fascination is Barbra Streisand's. Another is even more mystic—because her specific beauty has defied accurate description or analysis. While almost every part of her face taken separately—her forehead, chin, nose—seems unrelated to the others, together they achieve the impact that is Sophia Loren—right between the eyes.

It *is* those eyes—huge, slanting pieces of amber that seem to hold a glowing life of their own—that hold the key to the face.

Sophia has, of course, followed the beauty rule to maximize the most, and has concentrated on those remarkable eyes. Even to the point of having them opened up to a still wider slant.

As we can see, a face is divided into several parts, like Caesar's Gaul, even though having six instead of three. And it is not the separate parts, but the composition of those parts, that makes the living result.

51

But for most of us, too far a deviation from the ideal is not a pleasing result. To bring the individual framework more into line with the ideal is the aim of *all* aesthetic surgery—whether it be the face, the buttocks, the breasts, the thighs, or any part of the human organism on which nature has shown her imperfections.

Keats' classic "Beauty is truth, truth beauty" is followed by the less often quoted "that is all ye know on earth, and all ye need to know."

Quod erat demonstrandum.

CHAPTER 5

Face Lifts: Mini and Maxi

YOUTH passes, but beauty has no age.

Surgery to improve the face has already become such an accepted part of our life style that there is no longer the aspect of some sort of magic—of transforming a 55-year-old into looking twenty-five again. That's not magic, it's not very well adjusted wishful thinking. Anyone who wants to wipe out thirty years of living needs some self-examination before looking for a plastic surgeon.

That isn't the case with the preponderance of people—men and women—who do feel they are ready for, and *need*, some improvement of the face they are facing the world with. The question is not generally "How young will I look?" but "How long will it last?"

They do not necessarily equate looking better with looking younger, although one does result in the other. You *become* that person you see in the mirror when you get up in the morning: good to look at, able to function without the hangups of deterioration and to make the most of what your life has to offer.

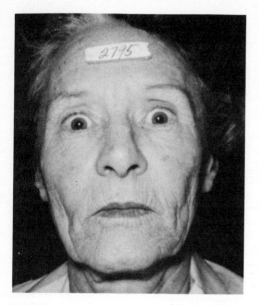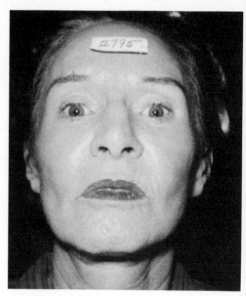

62-year-old woman who underwent blepharoplasty and rhytidoplasty, plus eyebrow lift, followed by chemical face peel four weeks later. Results at six months.

How long will it last? The result of a face lift is qualitatively and quantitatively as long as the patient lives. Analogously, take the case of twins who, say, die at age 60. If one had had a face lift at 40, she would have been the younger looking one all along. The years never do quite catch up.

But there is much more than the physical aspect involved. Sometimes a patient expects a miracle, and sometimes a seeming "miracle" does take place.

There is no doubt that very often what prompts a woman to get a face lift, hopefully, is to get a man in her life.

The face lift itself doesn't really make her a new person—it only opens up the possibilities of her becoming a new person. Or rather it opens up possibilities of fulfillment within the person.

It isn't only the way you look in the mirror, but the way you feel about yourself as well. The reflection that comes back at you *must* influence the way you feel and therefore the way you act.

If you feel improved by the new reflection there, then you *are* improved. In the end, it isn't really the face that gets the man but the attitude inside the person wearing the face. However, the man who gets interested does have to get past the face before he gets to the attitude.

The real and basic worth of plastic surgery is in making it possible for the patient to realize her potential. And increasingly this goes for men too.

In our youth-oriented society, it doesn't really matter how young you are, but how you measure up.

When *Esquire* magazine printed that cover with the girl in the garbage can, the first flush of that "over the hill at twenty-one" nonsense was really taken seriously, even viewed with alarm. Tongue-in-cheek *or* serious, and despite our accelerated pace of living, there are definite signs that we are coming back to some semblance of sanity in realizing that experience has its own inestimable value. And that, although by the figures the population *is* growing younger, even "over thirty" is not really senile, after all, and that over sixty or seventy or even eighty can be productive years.

We are in an age when it is not the date on your birth certificate that is important, but the way you function. It will become a fact of life that the "natural" progression of age as we have known it will, at best, be conquered and, at the least, controlled.

Some of this will be biological, from within in improved health and heredity. Right now, however, the physiological is strides ahead of the biological in the accepted results of plastic surgery.

Already there are those women who, understanding and making use of its possibilities, say, "I couldn't do without it." To them, this is no less germane than to the woman who says, "I couldn't do without my false eyelashes."

Old conditioning dies hard, so there are still women who like to keep their cosmetic surgery their little secret. But the natural acceptance of having your face improved when it needs it is becoming so general that it will soon be considered no more "unnatural" than having necessary dental work done. Plastic surgery is becoming part of our life style because our life style dictates the necessity for it.

In this broader aspect, the question proceeds from "How long will it last?" to "How often can it be done?" The simple fact is that face lifts can be had several times. Scars can be cut out with each succeeding lift or whatever other work needs to be done. Scars, in themselves, tend to fade or can even be minimized by such processes as dermabrasion. As Miss Mae West succinctly and accurately characterized the face lift, "It's only skin you're getting rid of. If you need to—why not?"

Plastic surgery is, in every sense, a surgical operation, however, and I do not hold with any so-called five-minute miracles. A current (and I hope soon abandoned) example of this is the mini-lift. It would, in fact, be a five-minute miracle if it worked; the only trouble with it is that it doesn't.

The mini-lift took hold in London, where all things mini—from taxicabs to skirts—started and became part of our civilization. Working girls would visit a plastic surgeon on their lunch hour and "have it done"—and it didn't really take much longer than that.

What happens in this misnamed "little face lift" is that the surgeon removes a piece of skin from each temple inside the hairline, then closes the incision—*fini,* the instant face lift! No bleeding, no after-effects; you just leave and go about your business.

Immediately afterward the patient is apt to be very pleased with the results of this quick-change artistry. But it will last only until the swelling made by the surgery goes down: several weeks, a month if she is unusually lucky, then right back to the original. Easy come, easy go.

I have had career girls ask me, "But isn't it worth it, even if it's only for that special appointment when I *have* to look great?"

My answer to that is, "No, because you're wasting your money. You might as well tape up your face instead."

Tape, of course, is the old standby in show business for that instant "temple lift" for special camera or stage appearances, but is certainly not to be considered part of routine makeup. It can get messy—and embarrassing!

It is obvious that I am not of the "tailor" school of plastic surgery: the little tuck here, the stitch there. These can be very useful in the overall picture of what happens in a face lift, but only as a means to an end. Plastic surgery should be considered seriously and done completely to meet the needs of the individual patient.

When should one have plastic surgery? Some women, conscious of the necessity to preserve their looks, will consult a surgeon *before* anything is needed. They just want to be sure that everything is under control and that they're not letting anything go unchecked that *may* be developing.

One such woman, an actress who in later years turned career business woman as well, came to me to "check for elasticity of the skin." She is past 40, but she is one of the lucky ones. Her skin is finely drawn and of an excellent texture, fitted closely over a good skeletal structure. I reassured her that any women her age would be lucky to be in the same condition, and told her not to worry about anything for at least a few years.

Actually, she wasn't being foolish or overanxious, even though her mirror told her everything was all right. Many women younger than she is come to me to ask for face lifts, and the fact is that they do need some correction.

The problem is that the fatty tissues under the skin tend to atrophy; it is a degenerative process that can be noticeable at thirty or not begin until one is fifty. I hesitate to do a full face lift on anyone under or even just past forty—but there are other corrections that can be done to start keeping the status quo.

Even on the full face lift, however, it is better to start younger than older. To state it another way, it is easier to keep things in shape than to have to get them back in shape after a great deal of damage has already been done. A face lift at any time is going to be an improvement—but a face lift *in* time is a sort of training for the face. There is more resilience to the skin, and an early face lift can slow up the aging process. It never lets things go so far that

57

you go through a period of deterioration. It helps keep you the person you want to be, not one you will have to struggle to become.

From the surgeon's point of view, it is simply a matter of getting better results by doing the face lift when it is needed and not years later.

Even so, when a patient comes to me and asks, "What can I expect of my face lift?" I always tell her, "It depends. Mostly on you."

There are many case histories of face lifts, but your own will be as unique as your own individuality.

Who, ideally, gets the most out of a face lift? I would say the woman between forty-five and fifty-five whose skin has retained some of its elasticity and who has fairly good bone structure and not too much dermal fat—and who wants to get back her *own* looks, not some mental image she may have carried around in her mind for most of her life of how she'd *like* to look. If you have never been happy about yourself, a face lift is not apt to be the thing to make you happy.

My favorite patient is the one who said to me, "But doctor, is this going to change my facial expression? I mean, I have always *liked* the shape of my mouth; I wouldn't want that changed. I don't want people *not* to recognize that it's me."

This woman didn't want to be somebody else. She wanted to be herself, only a better self than she had come to be externally. She was thinking of the tight, mask-like look that is the result of some plastic surgery. But that fortunately is getting to be a thing of the past, as surgeons become more and more conscious of the individuality of their patients and use their skills to preserve it.

A face lift is not merely a surgical diagram. It is even possible, in the case of the woman who has never been happy about herself, that her features may turn out looking more like the way she always wanted them to.

Recently I saw a very fine but aging stage actress on television, and the only thing I recognized about her was the voice. She looked younger, all right, but her face was drawn so tightly that you could practically see the new superimposed over the old, like a mask that had slipped slightly. Perhaps if she had had the requisite surgery ten years earlier, it would have worked out better. Perhaps she had simply chosen the wrong man to do the surgery. Whatever it was, it seemed tragic that this famous face should have become virtually unrecognizable and the woman unknown until you heard the voice.

To reiterate, a face lift should be done for the person and not out of a medical book diagram. Even where the scar goes will be determined by the individual face. Sometimes it is best to make the incision inside the temples and not the more classic back-of-the-ears technique. Depending on the structure and needs of the face, that method also allows for a tighter pull. With some men, who until longer hair set in couldn't afford scars in their closely cropped temples, I will make the incision straight across the brow (this has the youthful effect of raising the eyebrow) and the fine scar blends with the skin. Sometimes scars can be engineered simply to hide inconspicuously in a fold of the skin.

Contrary to vague impressions about the face lift, there is no cutting of muscles but only a cutting away of the outer skin, that hanging, sagging surplus. Other than that, the face lift can vary as much as the individual needs, and the surgeon's technique.

A full face lift is the plastic surgery process in which the facial skin and some of the neck skin are separated from their muscle and tissue, then pulled up and back. The excess skin—sometimes inches of it—is cut away and the incision closed.

Classically, the full face lift starts with an incision at the temple, in the hairline, then proceeds down around the front of the earlobe and back up under the hairline, winding up at the nape of the neck.

The variations on what happens in the process are too many to classify, depending on whether the problem lies in a double chin, sagging jowls, a turkey wattle, oversize cheeks. Even raising the forehead might improve the overall result, though this is rare.

How much is done sub-classic, you might say couture, depends on the man, his artistry, and even his desire to be thorough.

59

The professional word for face lift is *rhytidectomy,* from the Greek word for wrinkle, but oddly enough it seldom alone deals efficiently with all wrinkles.

The face lift will, of course, tend to smooth out wrinkles and even improve skin tone by heightening circulation. But there are some types of wrinkle that have to be dealt with separately. The surgeon can do something, for instance, about that wrinkling of the upper lip right after the lift, by using a skin peel solution. The "little things" that might have separately required the services of a plastic surgeon can usually be combined *with* the face lift and done while the patient is still anesthetized.

Having your skin refitted by plastic surgery can include a multitude of necessities, but if all you are concerned about is the skin itself, there are skin peels and sandpaperings and dermabrasions that sometimes can produce brilliant effects. On the other hand, if the plastic surgeon cares about the result *in toto,* he will not only give you a face lift that improves—without changing—the basic *you*, but he will be conscious of your skin texture at the same time.

If you really want to get the most out of what plastic surgery has to offer, then you will probably combine the face lift with a chemical skin peel three weeks later. This is treated in another chapter.

What really happens when you get a face lift? First, I want to see as much of you as possible *before* surgery. I want to study your face; hence photographs are taken, But more than that, I want to see how your face acts when you talk, smile, frown.

We will talk, and I will attempt to find out how you feel about it, why you want a face lift and what you expect from it.

Some women do not feel right about themselves and consequently will find it difficult to feel right about anything else. If you are one of these, I can foretell that your face lift will not live up to what you expect of it, and I will try to dissuade you. "Expectation" can take many forms, and a face lift can make a tremendous difference in making new things possible, but it cannot solve other problems not related to it.

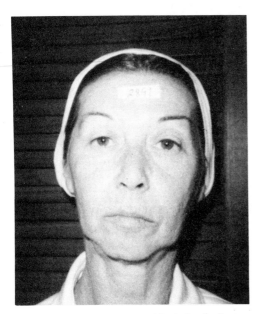 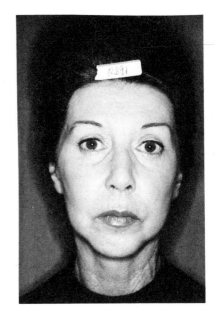

This lady had a renovation: eyes,
face lift, chemical peel, and chin.

If you are not at the proper weight, I might suggest that you put off surgery until you have lost some weight. The more weight lost, the more skin sag and therefore the more the "lift" accomplishes. Conversely, if you lose your excess weight *after* surgery, there will be a resultant sag from loss of subcutaneous fat.

Let us say that, all things being equal, we set an appointment for The Day. It is likely, if there are no unusual factors, that I will give you a choice: you can either go into the hospital, or you can have the work done in the surgery in my office. Ninety percent of my patients elect the office.

You will be given a local anesthetic, under which the operation, if it is a standard face lift, will take about an hour and a half. How you react depends, again, on you. Some people can have a tooth extracted and feel it really wasn't all that bad. With others, it can amount to almost major surgery.

61

You will, of course, feel no pain during the operation, from which you will emerge with your head bandaged in what looks like a white football helmet and gives you a sense of the importance of what you have been through.

After you have been driven home, you will of course be confined to bed and take medication to control any pain. You will be on a practically liquid diet for a few days, and incommunicado for the better part of a week, so far as talking is concerned—you will not spend much time on the phone with friends.

In two days, just like in the movies, the bandage comes off in the office. But unlike in the movies, the result is not the spirit-lifting scene where the hero opens his eyes and knows he has recovered his sight. Under those football helmet bandages the truth is that you are swollen black and blue. You won't be frightened, because I have warned you what to expect. But this is the point where you *don't* want to look at yourself. Most patients don't.

Now I give you a new and smaller bandage which can be covered with a head scarf. You go back home and mostly rest or catch up on your reading until four days later. Then you come back to the office. The eye stitches come out, the worst is now behind you, and the best is yet to come.

Now you begin to see the result. You feel the first thrill of the new smoothness, the refreshed, tightened, yes, *younger* face you're looking at. And it's all yours.

In two weeks hardly any scars show. There may be some slight visible indications, but there is something about facial surgery scars that seems to make them blend benignly with the skin so that they look natural and become unnoticeable.

Even those you might be aware of yourself, and that can be covered by combing the hair over them, somehow become so unimportant that you don't even bother to hide them. And the result is that you go *on* looking as if you've just come back from a vacation.

How long will it last? Again, it depends in large measure on you.

Mainly, the face will go on aging naturally from the date of the lift. But you will always be that much ahead of the game.

There are any number of ways in which a face can age or stay young. Some young girls have already damaged their skin more by excessive sunning than some women in their forties who haven't violated their skin texture in this way. Your physical condition can be another factor, and certainly your emotional one. The life you lead, and that includes your sex life, can keep your skin abloom with vigor or in the dullness of unfullfilment.

Right now, another gratifying type of plastic surgery that's done is the lid lift. This eye lift is something I combine with the face lift at times, but it is certainly not necessary to have a face lift to get the eye lift.

This produces a wide-awake, fresh, vital and appealing look that gives new meaning to the face. What it accomplishes primarily, of course, is to get rid of those eyebags and general puffiness that can suggest dissipation—or simply that your heredity gave you baggy eyes from birth.

The operation is called a *blepharoplasty,* from the Greek *blepharon,* or eyelid, and is one operation in plastic surgery that is almost easier to do than pronounce.

There are a number of variations on the *blepharoplasty,* involving both upper and lower lids, or perhaps only one or the other.

Eyebags are fat, herniating through the three separate pockets of fat in the lower lid and the two in the upper. By making an incision to remove the excess fat and excess skin at the same time, you remove the reason for eyebags and get smooth eyelids on top and serene smoothness underneath.

While the conventional procedure has been to go to the hospital, the eyelid operation is being done more and more right in the surgeon's office. In either place, it is generally done under a local anesthetic.

Although it is one of the simpler and more gratifying plastic surgery operations, it is more than getting your vitamin shot. You may be bandaged for around twenty-four hours, or you may not be, with the surgeon prescribing "blue ice," which is an eye mask filled with liquid which you chill in the refrigerator.

Your eyes will be swollen, of course, and for a few days you will look as if you might have walked into a door in the dark. By the fifth day, however, all the stitches will have been removed—the scar blending into the fold of the eyelid. For the underlid, the scar is hidden by the lashes.

The eyelid operation has nothing to do with your vision, although your vision will be tested beforehand as a precaution, but the possibility of any complication involving vision is not even considered remote.

Even in such a beautiful, almost freak-free operation there can be hazards. One former singing-acting star (who has never needed any breast augmentation, by the way) had her eyelids done with the result, due to the removal of too much skin, that the inner lining extended over her lower lids.

When she came to me, she was wearing dark glasses, which she insisted she even wore to bed. The corrective operation was far more difficult than a standard eye lift, but the result is now what it should have been in the first place.

It is possible to enumerate at least thirty "partial" face lifts that will take care of the lower face, the upper face, and unwanted anomalies ranging from accordion-pleated neck and dropped cheeks to dewlaps and thickened jawlines, all separately.

I cannot recall a single woman who has had this partial surgery who from hindsight did not say, "I wish I had had the whole thing done at the same time."

The full face lift is, after all, the only surgery that gets *both* the face and neck, in which it is possible to create the interrelated tension for taut smoothness in both, while treating the overall area as one.

This is not to say that the full face lift is itself the *only* satisfactory plastic surgery. The eyelid lift is a great case in point, and one which is frequently and commonly used on people in their twenties to get rid of those hereditary suitcases under the eyes. Those ubiquitous bags sometimes even figure in caricaturing the character in a face as much as the nose, as Duke Ellington himself will be the first to tell you.

Lately, a related operation to the eyelid lift has come into popularity, known as the eye*brow* lift. You might think this would be favored by patients who have developed the droop of maturity in this area, but that is not so. When it's gone that far, there is usually more to be done than the removal of excess skin under the eyebrows.

Actually, this repair is favored more by young people in entertainment, modeling and other related fields that keep them always in the public eye—for a vital, wide-awake, with-it look that is a built-in camouflage and belies how the performer may really be feeling.

This lift to the eyebrow is done under a local anesthetic, whether you have it done in the surgery or in the hospital. It takes about an hour, during which time the incision is made at the upper

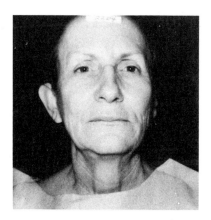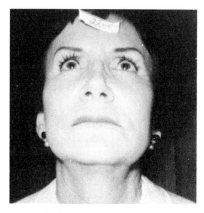

59-year-old woman who had blepharoplasty and rhytidectomy followed by a rhinoplasty three months later. Result after six months.

65

edge of the eyebrow and a bandage is applied only to the area affected. The stitches are removed after three to five days, the scar being concealed in the upper part of the eyebrow.

The eyebrow lift not only lifts the eyebrow and eliminates that hard droop at the outer eye, but it also tautens upper eyelids from wrinkled to smooth. It can even improve vision, in cases where eyelids have drooped enough to interfere with it. All in all, it can be a very satisfactory "little" operation, made to order for the needs of some faces.

And there is, of course, the now standard "temple lift," which takes in the droop around eyes and eyebrows, with the face lifted upward from within the hairline at the temple.

This operation too is easily done in the surgery under a local anesthetic without even any dressing to wear home. After surgery, gauze is pressed firmly to the incisions for several minutes; then the patient follows up with cold compresses at home. There will be swelling and some bruising, but recovery to "normal"—with the big plus of beauty, of course—within a few days or at most a week.

If I were asked what the ideal age is for getting the complete face lift, I would have to answer "when it is needed." The youngest face liftee I have known had it done at thirty-two and the oldest at eighty-seven.

These are, of course, the exceptions that prove the rule. In between, there is the fashion designer who at sixty-five has had plastic surgery three times.

The first time she was in her thirties. Her face was still all right, but she had always lived with deep nasolabial furrows running from mouth to nose—those lines the French call the lines of bitterness—and that is precisely how she felt about them.

The first plastic surgeon she consulted would not concede that the furrows warranted surgery. *She* felt there would be an improvement in her career if she improved herself and found a surgeon, who, as she puts it, "got rid of my hound-dog lines."

At this first face lift she did not have the eyes done, which operation came a few years later. Five years ago, almost twenty years after her first face lift, she wanted another.

66

How does she feel about facing a face lift again? "I wouldn't do without it," she says. It so happens that her other features—eyes (already done), mouth, teeth and, to take in the full picture, the legs—are so good that, in her case, plastic surgery was the only answer to getting rid of the imperfections that spoiled the perfections.

The surgeon's scalpel often provides that mysterious fountain of youth that the rest of the world marvels at. An actress who has been semi-retired for years, but who has been active in films again to some extent in recent years, is the marvel of interviewers who came to ask her for her secret of youth. She will never admit it publicly, but off the record she says, "Plastic surgery is something I cannot do without."

The legend of youth has attached itself to her for years, although she has not lived in Hollywood for a long time. Her secret, as given to interviewers, has always been the same: a serenity of spirit and existence, plenty of sleep, calm, moderation.

The legend goes with her serene look—a pure happenstance of nature achieved by her smooth, round young, forehead.

Although she had never before undergone surgery, she submitted to an unusual plastic surgery procedure: a scalp lift. It might, in a way, be called a "face lift" far back on the scalp, to maintain that serenity of forehead. It was done in the utmost privacy of a Swiss clinic, with security measures that required a scenario-like plotting. Having faced her first such venture with the worst fears and misgivings, once it was behind her, she realized that surgery is not something to be feared but to be thankful for.

One woman said to me, "My fifties have been the richest years of my life. I want everything about them to go on as long as possible." *She* had a total face lift a little over a year ago, and no one has ever suspected. She isn't startlingly changed, but her throat is neat; a small series of accordion pleats have vanished from under her chin; and her face is fresh, vital and good to look at.

But basically she looks like the same woman before the face lift. It wasn't a matter of adding something, but rather subtracting the unwanted. It's a situation in which those close to her would say, "You're looking so great these days. What have you done to yourself?" without really stopping to wonder about it.

It's the classic academic situation of *good* plastic surgery.

And when I see the personal exultation that is part of it—the surge of the spirit, the vitality of hope even *before* surgery—I know that all is not vanity but reality.

CHAPTER 6

Breasts: The Naked Truth

HAVING your breasts improved by means of plastic surgery isn't wholly a twentieth-century phenomenon. Medical history relates that in 1600 Durstan (a household name, of course, even among surgeons) reported a first attempt at a mastectomy to correct prolapsed breasts.

Nothing further seems to have been offered on the subject for 200 years, until Velpeau (another household word requiring, among surgeons, no first name for identification) published his own experimentation with the mastoptosis around 1854, by which time, of course, the medical habit of publishing "papers" was coming into full flower.

Now, well over a hundred years later, mammaplasty is a technique of surgical aesthetics, making it possible to build the bosom to the ideal it should represent.

It would be astounding to learn how many of those beautiful forms surrounding us in our current breast culture were not born but made, that way.

That goes from the cocktail goddesses of Las Vegas to the screen goddesses of Hollywood. One of the most amusing lines in this ubiquitous breast augmentation was, in fact, heard in Las Vegas.

Bringing along the first course to a table, a waitress noticed that the drinks had not yet been served. "Didn't that cocktail waitress bring your drinks?" she asked in disgust, adding, "I'll curdle her silicone!"

With the means more and more available, it becomes the norm to use them—with the end result justifying the means. And it *is* the result, in the end, that becomes the reality. Was Galatea any the less real because Pygmalion had created her?

The new bodies seem to accept as a matter of fact having everything in its right place, but to take less room for it. Today's figure is unmistakably female, yet less spread out. The clothes that go over it seldom allow for the idea of underwear, as it used to be known, at all. They just hang at some self-conceived natural angle of unrestrained rightness.

The Beautiful People were the first to make it a cult in today's scene that you had just better shape up. They got the idea, of course, from the young, who can afford to belong to this cult. Our new kind of ageless person was not far behind and soon got with this new freedom and awareness of the body.

Replacing the old acceptance that a *lady* always wore a girdle, there is now something almost vulgar in the *need* for a girdle. As for the falsie—not only was it relegated to the status of the farthingale, but in the cult of the natural even the bra itself was dropped.

Suddenly, we seem to have developed (and that must be the right word for it) a kind of woman with a new concept of breasts not as a separate entity, falsie-filled out and propped up to some engineering principle, but part of her own body. Since a good eighty percent of American women have heretofore been flat-chested, that poses something of a mystery, even a miracle. But through the annals of time, women have had a mysterious means

70

of fitting into the figure demanded by their own era—the ultimate example of female mind over matter.

Have women suddenly grown better breasts in general? The young probably have. Better nutrition has made them taller and larger than their mothers. But the young have a natural advantage in the body department by the very nature of their firm youthfulness. Perhaps the difference lies also in the eye of the beholder and the new conditioning to thinking of the breast as a soft appendage to the body, not a jutting abutment.

But what about the female who has been a big girl for some time now, and now realizes that her breasts just don't measure up? Women still have to be reassured in their psyches, being women. And there is no one part of a woman that will so disrupt her psyche as the feeling that her breasts are inadequate. Breasts are equated with sex. They are the part of her body that symbolizes her femininity in every way—to herself, to her lover, to the world.

And yet the female breasts, of all body organs, display the greatest variation of size and form and vary the most at different periods of the woman's life.

The moment of truth came not long ago when women removed the proppings, paddings, suspensions and whalebonings that were accepted as part of the feminine mystique. Now that the Merry Widow is out and skin is in, the bosom has to meet fashion's demands on it.

If fashion has dared the unveiling of the real breast—from see-through tops to minuscule bikinis—then the woman has to be woman enough to live up to it. Again, she becomes the product of her age.

This is all the more remarkable when you consider that, despite its own variations in the same woman—from puberty to pregnancy to beyond menopause—the breast does not lend itself to much change from outside influences.

Its size depends on the amount of body fat deposited in that cutaneous appendage known as the breast. Since it contains no muscle tissue, exercise cannot really make the breast larger. Good

71

body tone will automatically reflect itself in the bosom as well. And exercise, while it isn't going to make a 36 of a 32, will help, as exercise helps any part of the body, to tone and make it achieve its optimum.

Of course, even the breasts are dependent on the rest of the body. A slouchy posture will certainly make introverts of them rather than extroverts. And if you have reason to be self-conscious about your bosom, slouching is not going to help; it can only make things worse.

In this age of the nude ideal, it isn't surprising that we are also arriving at some psychological clues to the breast ideal. One is that breasts reward the woman with an awareness of them as part of her feminine body. Regardless of their shortcomings, she needs to consider them as such and make the most of what *is* there. Why, indeed, should breasts be made into a rigid ideal of some sort any more than a nose?

This is the new breast principle—and hooray for integration!—of seeing the breasts properly as part of the body they come with, not as separate entities that exist with a special label on them.

But aside from heredity, hormone levels, and the pure luck of what you were born with, there is the method that eliminates anything less than positive by simply creating a lasting, satisfactory bosom that presents none of the "natural" problems indigenous to the female. To this end, plastic surgery has eliminated, along with breast imperfections, as much psychic trauma as perhaps any psychiatrist's couch.

Mammaplasty (plastic surgery on the breasts) is considered not only safe but fairly foolproof as well. By this means, too large breasts can be reduced and reshaped, too small breasts can be augmented, and the sagging (ptosis) conditions that develop with years or from childbirth can be permanently corrected.

Breasts can be enlarged, lifted or reduced to appear perfectly natural, both to the look and the touch, and functionally as well. Mammaplasty in no way interferes with any of the natural senses or functions, even to nursing and breast examinations.

72

Breast surgery is almost always associated in the mind with augmentation, although enlarging is actually the simplest form for the surgeon to deal with. To me, it is breast reduction that presents a geometric challenge. It is also, from a physical standpoint, the most worthwile to do.

If anyone wants to find out how it feels to be *over-endowed*—a condition that has not been properly understood at all in our breast-conscious age—I have a 10-pound halter in my office that I hang around her neck. This instant realization of how it *feels*—my patients can't wait to get if off—to carry around this excess hanging weight is compounded by the awareness of other miseries. These can range from backaches, stooped shoulders and the difficulty of sleeping comfortably, to chronic cystic mastitis (a painful reddening of the breasts during menstruation and pregnancy, which seems to dispose a tendency to develop malignancy).

Correcting macromastia (overdevelopment) is more pathological

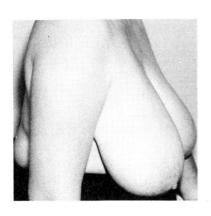

34-year-old female with mammary gigantism. Result in one procedure.

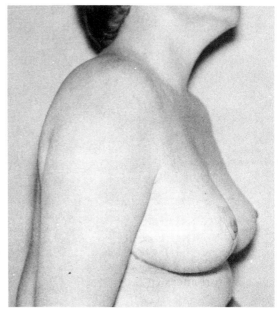

73

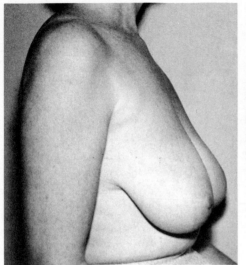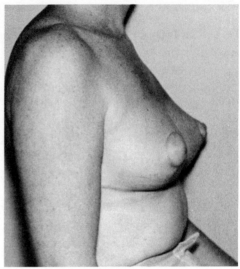

Reduction mammaplasty—40-year-
old female who had chronic backaches. Underwent a reduction mammaplasty. Result at four months.

than cosmetic surgery, and insurance companies recognize it as
such. It is, in fact, reconstructive surgery; therefore, it is to me the
breast operation that is most challenging and the most rewarding.

It represents a geometric challenge because the surgeon must
first destroy the contour of the breast as it exists and rebuild it, as
in the case of gigantomastia in a 29-year-old girl who, when I saw
her, had breasts extending below the level of her umbilicus.

This girl had gone from wearing a 34-c to a 40-dd brassiere in
the course of three years, during which time she had gained
twenty-seven pounds, from 108 to 135, and from merely large
breasts to a true gigantomastia. There were no hormone dis-
turbances; it was simply a case of undue fat deposit. And along
with it came severe emotional disturbance, feeling grotesque and
embarrassed, brassiere strap discomfort, chronic neckache, and the
necessity to have her clothes made to her measurements.

Reconstruction, with nipple transposition, resulted in sym-
metrical, mature, and only slightly pendant breasts with a planned,

natural, skin brassiere achieved in surgery. The nipples lost none of the erectile function and tactile sensation. The major scar lay in the submammary fold, hidden by the overhanging breast. The patient's postoperative course was uneventful, her brassiere size now being between 36 and 34-c.

Each case is a highly individualized one, much more special than that of enlargement. And that reminds me that most women with oversize breasts are just the reverse of their less endowed sisters—*they* want them small.

This, of course, is the over-reaction to the condition they have had to live with. The cosmetic result, aside from the highly important mental and fringe benefits, is that the woman now has the breasts she might have asked for, if she had had a choice in the matter. Is there scarring? Yes, a considerable amount. Is it worth it? Ask any macromastia victim who has been liberated. As for our 29-year-old *gigantomastia* victim, what she said after surgery was, "I don't know what to say. Except it's like being reborn."

What causes such a grief-making condition? Sometimes an endocrine imbalance or heredity. It can develop as an aftermath of pregnancy, or it can begin at puberty. In the latter case, the sooner corrected the better, as is obvious, and it can be done as young as thirteen.

Aside from the many "normal" activities—partaking in sports, even choosing clothes—that can become traumatic problems to a young girl with grossly oversized breasts, there is her relationship to boys. Breasts are part of her entire sexual adjustment; if they are too large or too small, the female may have a psychic inadequacy that she can be liberated from.

Men and boys—even at puberty—develop breasts, in which case any size is oversize. In the male, it is called *gynecomastia,* and it has nothing whatever to do with his masculinity. But it can cause embarrassment. It can be due to the glandular malfunction, and in a young boy it may disappear in a few years. It can occur with obesity, when fat develops everywhere, or, like Topsy, it can "just grow" as part of the physical makeup.

75

Breast reduction—or, in this case, the word is really elimination—in the male is far simpler than in the female, which seems only fair.

The operation can be done in an hour and a half under a local anesthetic in the office surgery—or the patient can elect to have a hospital stay of up to 5 days, until the bandages are removed and he is as good as new.

Either way, the procedure is the same: the incision is made around the nipple in the areola, the fatty tissue removed, and the incision sutured. There is not even a scar to remind him of his former emotional and physical disturbance.

Breast surgery includes correcting any kind of individual malformation from too much to too little—with variations in between, such as correcting the size of one breast to match the other, and postoperative correction to follow cancer surgery.

One of the underlying fears, in fact, of having breast augmentation is whether it will cause cancer. In a study made among *all* certified plastic surgeons in the U.S. in 1960, covering the previous ten-year-period, there was not a single case that indicated tumors

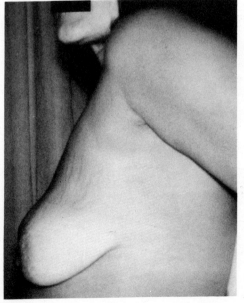
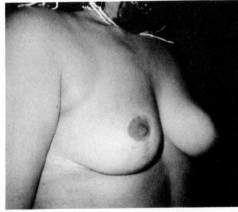

35-year-old female with drooping (ptotic) breasts repaired with one operation. Result at one year.

76

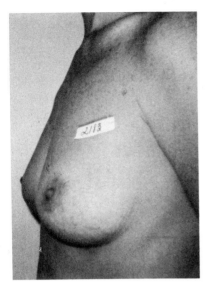
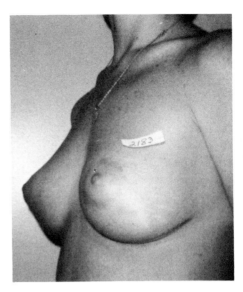

28-year-old female had repair of
post-partum drooping of breast.
One year after augmentation mammaplasty.

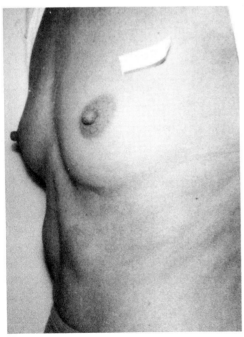
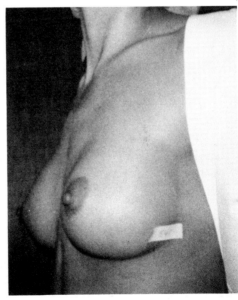

31-year-old female following augmentation mammaplasty because of
failure in proper development in
adolescence.

or cancers due to implants. On the plus side, because the implant goes in back of the breast tissue, the breast itself is more readily accessible to cancer checkups and biopsies.

The subcutaneous mastectomy, as cancer surgery is called, is done with the same silastic sack of silicone implant as for regular augmentation—except that in this case the entire breast has been cut away, along with the pectoral muscles and the lymph glands in the arm pit.

What it amounts to, then, is removing the skin and refilling it with the silicone sack. The procedure compromises the blood supply (because of the removal of the tissue and glands), and includes a high percentage of risk. In some cases, it is possible to retain only part of the nipple. But it is possible to remove all the tissue and glands and leave the pectoral muscle, inserting the implant behind *it*. This can be planned in the first stage—the removal of the breast—so that the muscle is left intact for the later implant.

I have had a special interest in breast cancer, and the sub-cutaneous mastectomy, because there is a family history of it from my great-grandmother to my mother, and an aunt as well.

In 1964 I began to work with Dow Corning on the silastic implant, following up my findings in a medical paper on the subject later distributed by Dow Corning. In 1966, at the San Francisco meeting of the American Society of Plastic Surgeons, I had an exhibit and a film of the operation. The general attitude was skeptical and not encouraging to the callow young newcomer (read whippersnapper) who seemed to be overreaching his place.

I have done some forty operations of breast replacement (not augmentation!), some following cancer surgery. About ten percent had complications, necessitating further surgical procedures; in only two cases were the complications serious enough to necessi-tate removal of the inserts. An article in *Look* in July, 1971, on the subject points out that the patient is usually more pleased with the breasts she gets afterward than the ones she had before, even though the procedure may not be for everyone.

The *Look* article says that plastic surgeons have done several

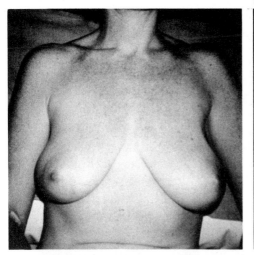
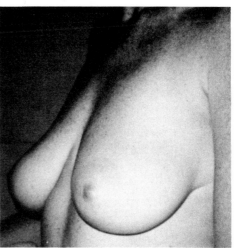
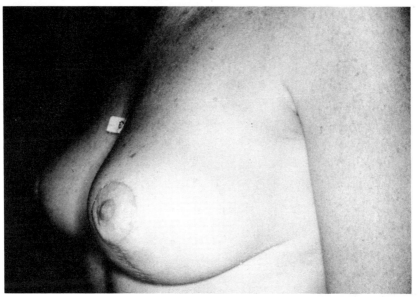

36-year-old female who had lifting
up of breasts and repair of asym-
metry. Result at three months.

thousand such operations, yet "the operation has gone un-
heralded; plastic surgeons fear to publicize it lest they be accused
of seeking personal publicity for profit."

I hope that the surgeon who is quoted here is somehow misquoted. With all the ethics involved in the profession, I cannot reconcile myself to reaching any sort of conscionable meeting between the fear of being accused of publicity seeking and leaving the millions of women who are affected and live in fear of being affected in ignorance of the truth that they need not be mutilated.

Mammaplasty is now so relatively simple as to be considered routine. The history of seeking to make women ideal in this wholly important area has come down from our early experimenter of the seventeenth century through the use of paraffin, sponges and fat cut from the buttocks and inserted in the breasts.

Experiments go on unendingly, but it is now considered both satisfactory and safe for a woman to have breast augmentation. For instance, I sometimes make the incision around the nipple, instead of, as is customary, in the inframammary fold, the crease under the breast; because then the scar becomes part of the areola and fades quickly.

The one lingering objection has been that a certain hardness

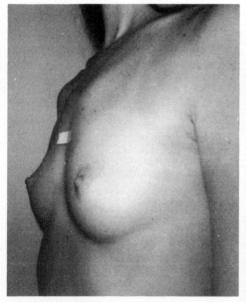

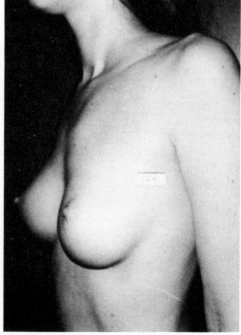

31-year-old female who had an augmentation. Result at six months.

sometimes develops if the tissues are stretched too tightly against the insert or there is postoperative bleeding. This is part of the surgical aesthetics of mammaplasty to fashion it so that this does not happen.

But the operation is now so well perfected that certainly there is no reason to wait on any future improvements. To reassure you further, it is a simple matter to open the incision and take out the transplant at any time. This is done if any complications develop, or (quite frequently!) when a patient decides she is still under-endowed or even over-endowed. And there are some eight sizes to choose from at the present time!

What happens in breast augmentation is that after a small incision in the crease under the breast (or around the nipple) is made, a bag of silicone gel or saline is then implanted in a pocket between the natural breast tissue and the chest wall. The sac unites with the tissue becoming a permanent, *natural* part of the body and therefore of the breast structure. It must have been what Keats had in mind when he sang that a thing of beauty is a joy forever.

What are the operative facts about mammaplasty? You can try on your implant in your own brassiere *before* surgery. And, yes, even a woman with virtually *no* breasts *can* achieve normal size.

The last photographs a woman will see of herself in her former condition are the ones taken just before surgery. They show only the upper torso, excluding the face.

Again, the patient can elect to go to the hospital or she can have the mammaplasty done in the office surgery under a local anesthetic. Let me repeat that under the local, the patient is not really *aware* of what is happening but is actually in a twilight sleep. I do not believe in suffering for suffering's sake, and I do not believe that it is good psychically for a patient to undergo any suffering in connection with plastic surgery.

This is a generally accepted thought; therefore the "forgetfulness" pill commonly associated with it. Actually the patient is kept under sufficient sedation not to have pain, even though there may be discomfort.

81

After the operation, which takes about an hour, the office even provides a new brassiere to cup each "new" breast with a light, firm bandage.

By the second day, the patient can be on a regular diet and resume a little activity—which I recommend as walking back and forth to the bathroom.

During the next two weeks you can read, sleep, get used to the idea of your *new* body image and enjoy being a Sybarite generally. As one patient put it, "Every time I look, I can't believe it's really me."

In the second week, the stitches come out in the office. You won't feel anything, and you will look for the scar. I will tell you it will fade, whether you find it in the nipple area or under the breast fold.

Not all bosom enlargements are done for actresses or go-go dancers or the nude Vegas chorines or young ladies hoping to make a reputation for themselves. Not by any means. As an example of how ubiquitous making the possible happen has become, here is a recent case history.

She was a young and very pretty Los Angeles Mexican lady of what we might call the lower middle class, with a husband and an assortment of children.

Everything was *muy simpatico* except that she was not amply endowed, and she knew her husband, dearly as he loved her, had a wistful longing that she might be. In fact, it was the husband who had heard about me and sent her to see me.

I assured her that she could, indeed, become everything her husband had dreamed of in this area. She returned to the office early one morning, had the surgery under a local anesthetic, and was transferred to spend the rest of the day in a recovery room adjoining the surgery. She had no one to take her home until her husband came to call for her after work. We had taken care of such an arrangement.

As is customary, he appeared Mexican style, *con su familia*. He had brought the children for all of them to bring *mamacita* home. She received them sitting up in a frilly bed jacket she had brought—just like all the "comforts" of a hospital.

When they surrounded her with affection and questions, she simply unbuttoned the jacket, to show them. Her husband gave a low whistle. Small pieces of tape under her breasts were evident; nonetheless the others stared in silent admiration. It was the oldest, a little boy of seven, who spoke the first words: "Madre Mia!"

The most satisfactory part of it is that the augmented breasts are as real as they look. The sensation remains normal, since the sensory nerve fibres have been untouched. It may be heightened, because of the lack of anxiety about inadequacy, and the fulfilled desire to give pleasure through the touch and feel of the full potential of womanhood.

While some women *know* how keenly they feel that their breasts don't measure up, others react differently. There was the patient who told me that she didn't understand her reaction to men until she had her breasts augmented. She enjoyed sex; what she kept asking herself was why when it came to the nitty-gritty, she found some reason to evade the situation. After the mamma-plasty, she told me how much easier it was to equate her feeling for sex with the feeling for a man.

It wasn't her chemistry that wasn't working. What she couldn't face up to was showing her inadequacy. Hence the man she could meet on all other terms became unattractive sexually to her.

The personal demand has now become a necessity for meeting the general demand for nudity. In St. Tropez, the local custom is nude sunbathing. You'd have to put even the word "bikini" in quotes. This is not only confined to day, because see-through anythings are the uniform of the night. Bras might easily be considered a collector's item.

And what they're doing in St. Tropez today—tomorrow, the world.

The realization of having breasts instead of hangups is a marvelous reality. The breasts are yours, a real part of your body, it *is* your body. And there's one thing more. They're not only for real, they're permanent and forever.

CHAPTER 7

About Miss Streisand's Nose:
The New Plastic Surgery

AS the standup nightclub comic had it, Barbra Streisand would do Jimmy Durante's life story when it was made into a movie. That's about the most far-out joke done to date about the celebrated Streisand nose, and had the comic's tastes run more to the classic, he might have substituted Cyrano for Jimmy, thereby at least lending a poetic overtone to his at-once amusing and questionable line.

Cyrano de Bergerac is, of course, the nose man of the ages, having glorified its meaning, its effects, its living, breathing influence on the wearer. Were Rostand around today in the Streisand orbit, it is unquestionable that he would paraphrase his own line to "a great nose indicates a great *woman*," with an assenting, sweeping bow from Cyrano himself.

The Streisand sloping profile, twin to Nefertiti's, is one of our natural wonders—a living work of art. It is to her credit that she had the awareness of self to make the most of it, and that she did not exchange greatness for conformity.

It is also to her credit that she has influenced the view of the nose generally. The small but flaring nostril, the nasal angle of 30 degrees fashionable in rhinoplasty, with a nasolabial angle of 90 to 95 degrees for men and 100 to 110 degrees for women, is no longer *de rigueur.*

The nose, I am happy to say, has progressed from the in-fashion *one* kind of nose that everybody wanted at the same time—"Give me a nose like Elizabeth Taylor's." Now there is the highly individualistic query: "What can you do to my nose to improve it but make it right for *me*?"

Not that there aren't a fair share of what I call nose neurasthenics around. There are the ones who have had 3, 4 and even 5 rhinoplasties—and I do not exaggerate merely to make a point.

Some people just go on seeking what they nebulously consider their perfect nose—and never find satisfaction. The dissatisfaction in these cases must be not with the nose but with themselves.

Because rhinoplasty has long been the most familiar of general cosmetic surgery, it would seem the simplest as well. To me, the "nose job" presents more difficulties than almost any other in the cosmetic field. This is not in the surgery itself, but in how you approach it. There are a number of *other* factors associated with having your nose changed.

First, even 1 or 2 millimeters (a minute fraction of measurement) can make a terrific difference in the final result. Second, there is the exact consideration of how to restructure the bone and cartilage so that there is neither too much or too little bridge.

Then, especially in the case of a large nose, you don't know how the skin is going to shrink, though that is still a factor that must be considered at the time of surgery.

A new nose takes about a year to set into its end result. Just after the operation, before the swelling subsides, it is most likely to seem the most satisfactory. Again, a nose that may seem too short to the patient at first may wind up exactly the right size.

I would say that ninety to ninety-five percent of my patients who have nose corrections are satisfied; my own satisfaction ratio is only about eighty percent. Real nose neurasthenics are in the minority. Most people who come out with a better looking nose are apt to be satisfied with the improvement, especially if they

86

have had a deviated septum and find they are now able to breathe properly. But a surgeon is constantly striving for perfection, and there are some things that virtually cannot be seen until afterwards, in how the nose itself reacts.

But *before* the fact, no nose can be considered in itself, but only as part of the entire face. There is such a correlation between the nose and the chin, for example, that one cannot be considered without the other. It is safe to say that seventy percent of nose corrections need some corresponding work done on the chin as well. Conversely, sometimes a chin correction is what is needed, and not a nose change at all.

This obviously leads us into all kinds of unsymmetrical combinations; the too long nose and the too short chin, now part of history as "the Andy Gump," the too prominent chin and the too short nose and other cases where nature has displayed a marked lack of artistry.

Which reminds me that if Barbra Streisand *had* had her nose remodeled, she probably would have had her chin remodeled at the same time, which prompts the thought that then there would be a *different* Barbra Streisand, and what a loss that would be!

Sometimes, however, there is the case where it is the nose, and the nose alone, that needs changing in order to release a new personality.

I can think of no better case in point than one of an appealingly pretty young girl who was changed into a smashing beauty.

Her nose tended to flatten, with not enough bridge and a bit too much nostril. It wasn't bad, really, as noses go, and more, it didn't really seem out of place in her face at all. That is what made the subsequent change so remarkable.

Remember, this was already a pretty girl, and the one feature that was less than desirable was absorbed quite easily by the generally good composition of her face. Her parents, by this time so used to seeing her with her natural nose that they couldn't visualize her with a different one, couldn't understand her determination to have her nose "fixed."

Nonetheless, she had been badgering them about it since she

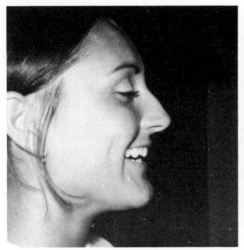
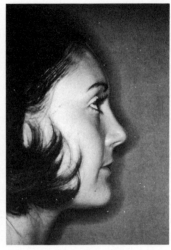

21-year-old female needed rhinoplasty. Result at five months.

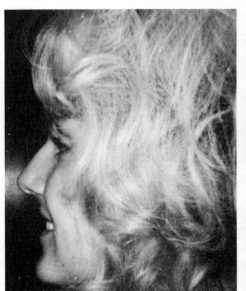
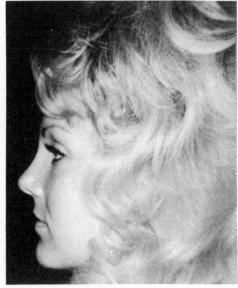

See what a nose correction did for
this 25-year-old girl. Right-hand
picture shows result four months
after operation.

was about age ten. They, who wouldn't have denied her anything they considered necessary to her well-being, simply listened with tolerance and the feeling that it was all a youthful whim she would outgrow. After all, this was a well adjusted child with no obsessions in other directions, and both sides had the unusual good sense not to press an issue that couldn't be resolved anyway until the late teens, the earliest time—unless there is some real malformation—for a rhinoplasty.

The issue never did come to a family crisis. When she was sixteen the girl simply began saving money out of her allowance, and at eighteen she came to me and, not bothering with preliminaries, said, "I have saved $400 to have my nose done. Will you do it for that?"

Her parents, who would have paid for it without question once they were confronted with the immovable fact that the time had come, agreed. Not with misgivings, but still with the sort of mental shrug with which the best intentioned parents sometimes indulge what they consider a youthful whim.

Her nose was the proper length for her face, so there was only the slightest cartilage manipulation to raise the nasal tip infinitesimally. All it really needed was a narrowing of the nasal pyramid and a trimming of the upper lateral cartilages on both sides—thus narrowing the nose and giving a more delicate flair to the nostril.

Changing her nose didn't change her psyche or the girl she actually was. But it did change the pretty girl with a somewhat flattened nose into a piquant, unmistakable beauty.

Of course, the wonder of this case is that, rather than being malformed, this girl's nose had seemed so naturally hers that what a change would do simply couldn't be visualized. Only *she* was female enough to sense it, and wise enough to know herself. As it turned out, she was not being headstrong—only determined enough to achieve what she wanted.

Of course, not all rhinoplasties (from the Greek *rhino*: nose) are such simple ideals of cosmetic surgery. There are malformations such as hooked and crooked and humped noses, saddle noses (depression of the bridge resulting from either congenital or acci-

89

dental causes), too long or too short noses—and combinations of those and others. Abnormalities vary from fractured noses to deviated septums (in which the mucous membrane interferes with breathing), and there are as many reasons for nose surgery as there are abnormalities. All deformities can be improved.

As we have seen in the previous case, the too-wide nostril and flattened bridge type of nose is not necessarily a racial characteristic and can be Caucasian as well as Negroid. Nor is the "new" plastic surgery for blacks as recent as it might seem. Weir (1892) described an operation for the correction of Negroid nostrils, consisting of the excision of a portion of the base of the nostrils, extending around the base to the area of attachment to the cheek.

There was later an improvement on this technique when Joseph, in 1931, and Aufricht, in 1943, reduced the area of excision to the base and floor of the nostril—the same method in general use today.

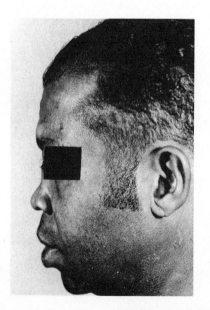 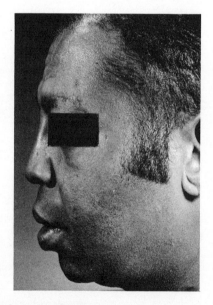

Saddle nose deformity secondary to infection. Treated with a bone graft from the hip. Result at one year.

90

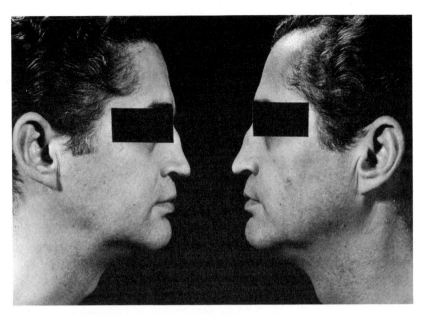

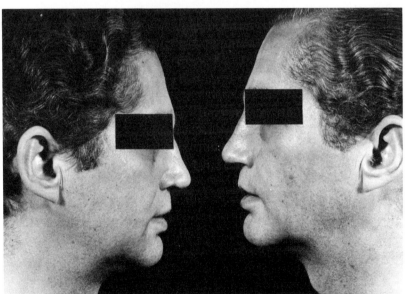

38-year-old man with nose damaged in accident. He had a rhinoplasty with a silicone insert to fix the profile.

91

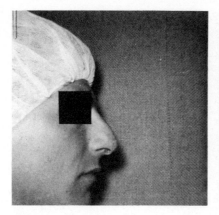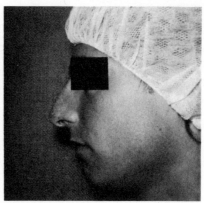

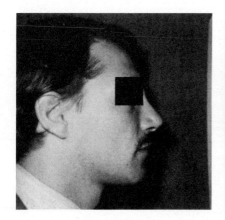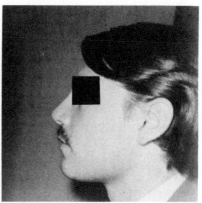

28-year-old physician who had accident and underwent rhinoplasty.
Result at four months.

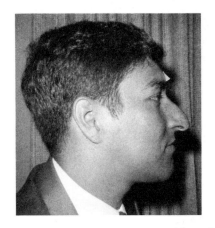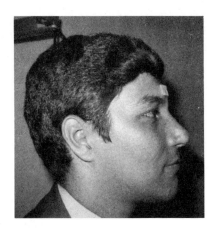

27-year-old male with large nose
had rhinoplasty and chin correction. Result at six months.

A Negroid rhinoplasty differs from the Caucasian in that it consists of taking out more tissue, usually of a coarse consistency, and considerable building up of the bridge with augmented cartilage. There is also the greater chance of keloids, or scarring, because of the natural skin consistency.

At the same time, it is also a very simple addition in symmetry to make the lips smaller. An incision is made on the inside, where it doesn't show, in the buccal mucosa (where the moist part of the inner lip meets the dry).

This presents more of a reconstruction job, but it is certainly well within the realm of possibility. In show business the black entertainer is as likely to have had cosmetic surgery of some type as his white counterpart. With the TV camera closeup moving in for those "pore shots," this becomes practically mandatory.

A part of the new plastic surgery is, for a fact, concerned with racial, or better still, inter-racial characteristics. Ethnic looks are getting to be accepted in the same way as are regional accents. The mid-Atlantic accent, homogenizing the best of both sides, becomes analogous to a physical homogeny of what is considered pleasing to the eye.

But unlike the already common Oriental eyelid operation, in

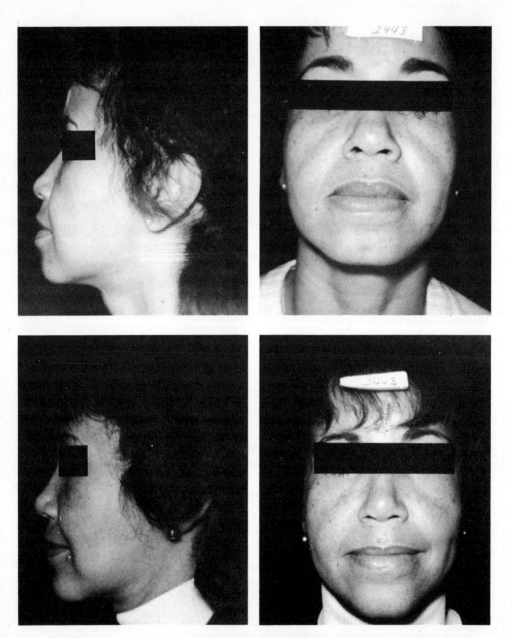

38-year-old woman who had a chin enlargement and rhinoplasty, as well as thinning of the lips in two separate procedures. One year post-operative view depicted below.

which a slit is made in the lid fold and the skin pulled upward to change the look to Occidental, there is no such typifying operation for Negroes.

One thing *is* sure, that more black people, like *all* people, are investigating and taking advantage of the possibilities of plastic surgery. And I find that what all black people care about are the same things that *all* people care about.

Black women are women, without the qualifying color adjective, with the same female hangups and desires and psychology. Black males are under the same pressure as their white counterparts to keep up by looking well and fit for their jobs.

Not all plastic surgery on black people is done on those in the entertainment world by any means. More awareness and affluence are bringing in more and more non-show-biz Negroes to the plastic surgeon's office. Do you know what the most popular operation is? It doesn't know any color. It's a face lift.

The nose, to return to this fascinating appendage, is the least static of the facial features. This member never stops growing or displaying a bent of its own, from the time, at 16 or 17, when it can be considered to have jelled, to the later date when it can assume the nobler proportions of living—from a bulbous tip to an accumulation of nodules and spider veins.

From W. C. Fields to several of our excellent present day character actors, it is apparent that they think too much of their proboscises to let any plastic surgeon fiddle around with them. In some cases, to have tampered with the nose would have been tampering with Providence—as in the case of the Great Durante.

Nonetheless, the nose has been fiddled around with by physicians since the time of the Egyptians. They packed the nostrils with lint covered with grease and applied external bandages. Hippocrates occasionally used tampons of sheep's lungs and a myriad of bandaging techniques to keep the member in place. Occasionally skeptical of their efficacy, he even had some patients hold the broken parts together with their hands.

He would probably be fascinated to see the somewhat newer techniques of today. More than any other surgery, I would rather see the patient have the nose correction done in my surgery and under a local anesthetic. We are familiar with the reality of the "bloody nose." A local anesthetic not only keeps the bleeding minimal, but allows for easier breathing.

All the general things I have said about office surgery and local anesthetics are especially pertinent in the rhinoplasty.

The operation will take around forty-five minutes, and after a few hours rest, the patient can be taken home and instructed not to talk too much. The bandages are removed in a few days in the office, then an adhesive applied for another few days.

There is some discomfort and there can be a great deal of bruising, right up to the eye sockets. Here again, conditions depend on the individual tendencies of the patient. Some will not bruise as much as others, but there *is* bruising. That part of it is relative, anyway, since in about a week or ten days normal life resumes no matter how little or how much one has bruised in the interim.

If the eyes are the spirit or the mirror of the soul, and the mouth reflects the emotions or the sensitivity, then the nose is said to be the symbol of character.

In famed instances, the nose has made the character. Dean Martin might not have made it with his old nose; certainly not in the sexy superstar image he has.

Then there are the elective ones. Karl Malden has kept what can certainly be called a supernose and it probably hasn't made any difference in his career as a fine actor; Liza Minelli had a bulbous nose, which she had "done," but it depends on what angle you are looking at it as to whether it is piquant or bulbous. Since she is Liza, it doesn't seem to make much difference.

But it's the exception that finally proves the rule. The influence of a superstar seems to have taken us out of the carefully constructed assembly-line noses of a few years back to the creation of a nose that suits the face—with all related factors, especially the chin and lips, considered in the final result.

Today's trend doesn't go in for those tiny noses almost too small to accommodate any bridge at all and that look as though there is no room to breathe through them. A number of glamour-pusses have precisely this kind of nose, and they're stuck with it. Smaller, you can do; larger, no.

It has come to be a matter of what is seemly, not what is foolishly chic. As Miss Streisand said of her own nose, and she couldn't have said it more aptly, "It's aesthetic."

CHAPTER 8

Body Sculpture: Cosmetic Surgery All Over

THE BODY corresponds to the face in developing the insulting sags of age. As upright animals, the entire organism is constantly fighting the law of gravity—always waiting to fall. It's that immutable law that what goes up must come down.

But just as all parts of the head and face can be corrected—from cleft palates to prognathic jaws—the indignities visited on the body can be cured as well.

Cosmetic surgery of the *body* somehow seems a great deal more removed from reality, perhaps because it covers larger areas; perhaps because we have become accustomed to the idea of facial cosmetic surgery for much longer. Actually, both are now common parts of the plastic surgeon's repertoire.

Aside from mammaplasty, which is fast catching up with the face lift as generally accepted plastic surgery, the most common body sculpturing is the stomach lift. And there are about ten different variations of the stomach operation to remove that excess sag and drag. My own most common procedure is to make the incision below the bikini line—where it is easiest to "lose" the scar in the pubic hair—cut out the excess fat and skin and pull up the remainder into a taut, smooth stomach.

The stomach can be called the fat bank of the body. It is not only capable of, but subject to, the storing of fat. Add to this the prevalent human predilection for overeating, and the result is trouble. The fat causes sag, and the combination is a common distress of our food-loving but body-conscious society. Dealing with it is fast becoming common procedure, because the human body is so subject to this aesthetic "stomach trouble."

Actually, there is no set reason for the pendulous overhang of the midsection that both men and women are subject to. Many times, weight has nothing to do with it or even the loss of elasticity that comes with time. I have corrected an obvious little paunch on an otherwise *thin* girl of twenty-five.

It seems to come down to a question of heredity, how much elasticity there is in your muscles and how lucky you are in various other ways. Childbirth, for example, is one of the ways a formerly trim stomach can come to sag. Once subjected to the indignities of stretching—whether from child-bearing or over-eating—the stomach skin may lose elasticity and may not easily snap back.

Overindulgence, underexercising, and over-age are the greatest contributing villains to stomach sag. But it is also true that there are cases where no amount of exercise or diet will correct skin inelasticity or encourage certain fatty deposits to dissolve or overcome hereditary tendencies.

Sometimes dieting will only make an already prolapsed stomach more unsightly. The fat is gone, but now the skin remains hanging with nothing to take up the slack.

The pendulous abdomen can be a hazard in almost all of life's activities—from finding clothes to sex.

But most of the time, both physical and psychic difficulties can be cleared up with the reshaping of this unwanted protuberance. There are case histories associated with every stomach lift which tell that other difficulties have been lifted at the same time.

The stomach *lift* actually touches no internal organ; it is only the excess fat and tissue and outer skin that are removed. It is not

100

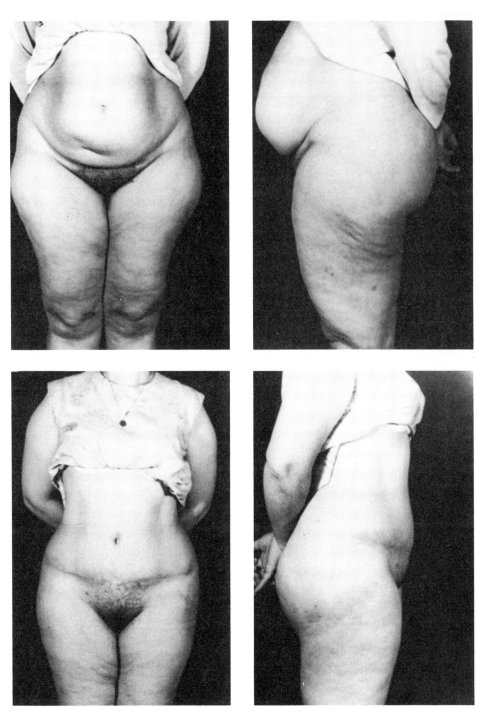

40-year-old woman had abdominal
and thigh lift. Result at six months.
(Courtesy of Dr. Marcos Szpilman)

considered a major operation—or even a serious one—under ordinary conditions.

It is performed under a general anesthetic, with a tight abdominal dressing following surgery that the patient wears for several days, with the stitches being removed a few weeks after that.

The scar, depending on the patient and the amount of surgery involved, may be slight or extensive. Sometimes it may be so involved that the patient will "lose" his or her navel—in which case the surgeon may improvise a fake one.

But the latter occurs only with cases of severe obesity or other abnormalities. The general stomach lift is usually done with what I call the under-bikini line, in which the scar is well below the navel, sometimes lost in the pubic hair, and almost always small. If the scar is bothersome to the patient, it can later have a "revision" in which the scar tissue is cut out and a finer line results.

In almost every case, when the patient is asked, "Which would you rather have, the scar or the sag?" there is never any contest.

Nature just seems to have designed the human body with most of its fat storage below the waistline. Next to the stomach, that unwanted fat seems to get most permanently attached to the thighs, especially in women, and after that, the buttocks.

Common *trochanteric lipodystrophy* has, in fact, nothing to do with glandular disorder or overweight. It seems simply that a woman is heaviest between her waist and her knees, creating the stomach-hips-buttocks syndrome.

What's more, the aesthetic imbalance of fat in this area is also a biological mystery; it is the most resistant to ordinary exercise and diet. How many women have remarked, when losing weight, "But I seem to be losing it all in my breasts!"

Just as in the stomach, *lipodystrophy*—or fat deposits—of the thighs can also be accompanied by sagging or loose skin, a condition that occurs in men as well as women.

Flabbiness, "dewlaps," whatever name this condition goes by, the indented dimpling of the hanging folds of the thighs and the corresponding droopy seat that goes with it, used to cause consternation at bathing suit time. Now, with the closeness of the world and more leisure practically eliminating the seasons, it causes consternation all the time. And there is no season at all on the growing awareness of the human body as it is, without the social disguises.

The improvement of saddlebag hips, those flaps on the outside of the upper thighs, has come to be generally known as the riding breeches operation.

The thigh lift raises the flabby fold of the inner thigh. In either case, or in both, if necessary, it is just as simple to include a buttock lift at the same time, so that the entire area undergoes a scalpel sculpture.

The incision is a line like an inside trouser crease—with the skin pulled upward and backward from the inner thighs around to the buttocks, the suture line being made in the fold of the buttocks. The line of the incision over the outer thigh and the buttocks is not visible in a bathing suit. The inner thigh incision will be, but the scars tend to fade with time and, as in the stomach lift, can be subject to revision.

The correction of thigh and buttock symmetry has progressed

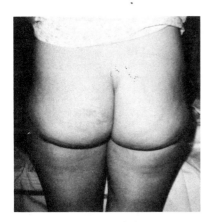 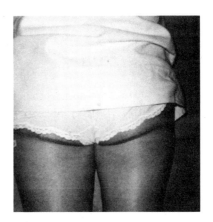

Saddle breeches deformity—29-year-old female with riding breeches deformity underwent a buttock and thigh lift. Result at six months.

103

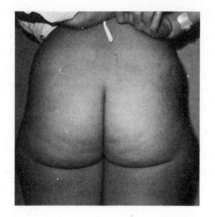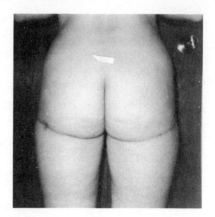

25-year-old female had a buttock raise and repair of riding breeches deformity. Result after four months.

in the past ten years to become a major improvement over the original "riding breeches" operation, which left long vertical scars and did not tend to correct what I consider a far more prevalent problem—the flaccid inner thigh. Now the one operation corrects the whole area, and with far more skillful suturing techniques.

The thigh-buttock lift does require hospitalization, and is done under a general anesthetic. Generally it entails about two-and-a-half hours. The patient is able to lie on her back the same day, to walk comfortably after four days, and to sit down without discomfort in about a week.

Generally there are no undesirable aftereffects, such as swelling. The lymphatic circulation is not interfered with by this operation.

The arm lift is far less common than the thigh lift at the present time, although it can be considered as corresponding surgery. Actually, the same condition of the upper arm obtains as of the inner thigh—with that unattractively dappled hanging fold of skin looking as if it had disassociated itself from the rest of the limb and were looking for some place to go.

A number of plastic surgeons will still not do an arm lift,

claiming there is no way of hiding the scar. But the operation is both safe and simple. It can be done under a local anesthetic, taking about an hour and a half for both arms in normal circumstances. The patient can go home right after the operation (or the next day, if it is done in a hospital) and will have the stitches removed in the office in about a week. There is no pain associated with an arm lift, and the scar is under the arm, in the least obvious part of it.

So many arm lift patients are pleased with the results that it is surprising that some plastic surgeons still hesitate to do it. A woman who has had such an operation comes into the office happily wearing a sleeveless dress. What scar there is she considers a welcome exchange for the former flabbiness of her upper arms.

Like all cosmetic surgery, this is an operation of choice, and I have yet to have an arm lift patient who did not consider it one well made. "So what?" asked one woman, "who's going to look *under* my arm for a scar?"

This attitude toward *all* cosmetic surgery scars is the one I like best to hear. It is absolutely true that the word "scar" causes a far worse mental reaction than eventuates in the reality.

Scars, too, become part of us, and with familiarity soon become "invisible." At first, the patient thinks everybody sees the scar—wherever it may be—that she is so conscious of. Before long, she finds that no one else pays any attention to it. By the time it has faded, it has faded in her mind as well.

I know a handsome young man (he looks rather like Robert Stack) who was in a very bad automobile accident in Nashville. He had about thirty stitches taken in his scalp and face, and at the time, he asked the doctor doing the suturing, "I know this is going to leave scars. What plastic surgeon do you recommend when I get back home to Hollywood?"

The doctor wisely told him, "You can't do anything about the scars for at least six months anyway. And you don't know what they'll look like. Why don't you just wait and see?"

It is now a year since the accident. The young man combs his hair over the scalp scars. As for the scars on his face, he is one of

105

the lucky ones. He has the fine skin that doesn't scar badly. "Why," he says, "nobody seems to notice them. Why should I bother about it?"

The point is that scarring is relative. It is the operation itself that is important in the final result. This is expressed rather well in a rather bad joke about the indignities of aging. The female comics adore it, and it goes, "But what *really* hurts is when people say to you, 'Your stockings are wrinkled'—and you're not wearing any!"

Yes, leg formation can be improved, too, as in the thigh and arm lift. But at present it is done more as necessary reconstructive surgery than as cosmetic surgery. Those scars, again. And on the lower leg they can be obvious.

On the theory of compensation, which always seems to work, there are dividends accompanying body sculpting as well as what scars there may be.

For one thing, no surgeon is going to operate to smooth and tauten body areas without the patient's weight being at par. I have had patients who have dieted for the better part of a year before they were ready for the stomach lift.

Once this weight is off, and once the body has been sculpted into that hoped-for shape, even a glutton is sure to lose his appetite rather than spoil the transformation. So one benefit reacts on the other. The body that becomes more beautiful on the outside is very likely to become that way inside as well.

Having cosmetic surgery of the body is about where face lifting was some ten years ago, with the exception of breast surgery. *Young* women are, in fact, thinking in terms not of having "something" done, but of "having the body done."

One such jet-setter of thirty-three checked into a Swiss clinic for a mammaplasty and a stomach lift. She didn't need anything else, but when she emerged in ten days she didn't need anything. As she told me when she got home, she was as perfect as she wanted to be, with "no hangups about the way I look to influence the way I *feel.*"

CHAPTER 9

The Face Peel:
Getting a New Skin

FACE peeling—until just about yesterday—had about it something of the aura of an illegal abortion. Medically, both were in just about the same class; today both have been legitimized.

Face peeling—or getting a new skin—is both the newest "phenomenon" of our avid youth culture and one of the oldest beauty practices in history.

Ancient formulas for getting a new skin are written in Hebrew in the Talmud. It is credited to Cleopatra that (along with all the myriad other avant-garde beauty practices she is credited with) she used hot bricks to burn off the old top layer of skin. Skin peeling was, indeed, practiced by the Egyptians and Babylonians.

Yet the skin peel of today has not been as available as cosmetic surgery itself, nor has it had the publicity. Up until just about yesterday it was shrouded in mystery, attended by the atmosphere of old wives' tales. Written stories have run from exposé to endorsement. With plastic surgeons, it had about as much scientific dignity as a cabalistic ritual.

It is only since the early 1960s that the technique of skin peeling with chemicals was even dignified with a medical name: chemosurgery.

In the space of about five years, its status in medical journals went from the extreme of the horror piece, *The Face Burners* (dealing with peeling done by non-medical practitioners), to the statement of the Committee of Cutaneous Health and Cosmetics of the American Medical Association itself in 1966.

In the AMA paper titled: *Superficial Chemosurgery,* the first paragraph states:

"For more than a hundred years dermatologists have used chemical cauterants mainly to treat small, benign neoplastic lesions and chronic inflammatory patches." The paper progresses to: "Recently extensions and modifications of chemical cautery have been used for cosmetic improvement of actinically damaged, aged and wrinkled skin."

That is a capsuled summation by the AMA of the progress or status of the chemical skin peel: that "actinically damaged, aged and wrinkled skin" has a way of turning into a brilliant new bloom—on men as well as on women.

On the other side of the picture, the dangers attributed to having a face peel have been legion. The basic fact remains that the means of exchanging prunes for peaches is by a chemical burn, whereby the outer skin is actually burned off by an acid, usually phenol (whose common name is carbolic acid), an agent not meant to be played around with.

This scary path to beauty has a history of scarring, blotching, and lesions of the skin—as well as internal damage from bodily absorption of the chemical resulting even in purported deaths.

The practitioners of the face peel *before* plastic surgery dignified it as a cosmetic process makes a fascinatingly dubious history.

There is perhaps a mystic corollary to be drawn from the fact that there has been a flourishing colony of face peelers in Florida, where Ponce de Leon sought the legendary fountain of youth. These fonts of operations came to be known as "wrinkle farms." Self-taught lady exponents of the art have become famous, as well

108

as notorious, also in Southern California—a place that made Ponce the also-ran in the pursuit of youth.

It is almost as mysterious as the former shadowy status of face peeling itself that, although almost all states have laws against face peeling by non-medical persons, these practitioners exist—and still keep springing up from California to New York.

Within plastic surgery itself, face peeling has acquired its own legends. It is even rumored among the humor-mongers in the profession that the real reason plastic surgeons took so long to legitimize the face peel was that they didn't know how to do it.

From there, it is only a step to the story that it was a plastic surgeon who first persuaded a lady practitioner of the art in Florida to sell her secrets to him. Probably under a full moon, with accompanying incantations.

What the plastic surgeon has been automatically opposed to is face peels done by face peelers. The peeler is dealing with toxic agents that can produce burns or scars or kidney damage, for which medical supervision is a prime requisite. Perhaps it is closer to the truth to say that the surgeon was practically forced to legitimize face peeling because of its bizarre and hazardous history in non-medical hands—and the peelees who took the risk, regardless.

Today, plastic surgeons use chemosurgery without trepidation, and mainly as an adjunct and a brilliant finish to plastic surgery. My own technique is to do it right in the office surgery under a local anesthetic. The agents most commonly used are phenol or trichloracetic acid. I prefer about a 50-percent phenol solution, with a tape mask, because the tape allows the phenol to penetrate deeper.

Incidentally, that is the basic "secret" of the solution used in face peeling—something any pharmacy can make up. The application, and the possible results, during and after application, are something else again.

The patient returns to the office in forty-eight to seventy-two hours, at which time the tape is removed, and is given thymol iodide powder to apply for three days, three times a day. An easy way to do this is to fill a salt shaker with the powder and sprinkle the face liberally. A crust forms after a few days, which should be left undisturbed until the sixth or seventh day following the chemical painting and taping. At that time, the crust is lubricated with vaseline ointment and begins to separate and peel off. Back to the office on the seventh day for general checkup and instruction on procedure.

The worst time would seem to be the first twenty-four hours. The burning sensation is controlled by medication, and because movement can crack the mask, food intake is limited to liquids (which allows for an unexpected dividend of some weight loss!).

In about two weeks you're able to face the world again, with your literally new skin a very rosy hue. There is apt to be some later disappointment. For the first few months after the peel the skin is plumped out—actually by edema or swelling—so that lines become invisible. Some of them may return when the contours settle back to what they will be normally. If necessary, the process can be repeated in twelve weeks.

What happens in a face peel is the coagulation of the external layer of skin, which removes the dry, withered and blotched epidermis. There is, along with this, some constriction of the skin. Although this means that there is a tightening of the skin along with the new, baby-soft quality of it, the current consensus of plastic surgery is that the face peel alone will not be too successful on sagging jowls, droopy chicken necks, suitcases under the eyes, or any such conditions which really require surgical correction.

But where plastic surgery is indicated, it is now being followed up more and more with a face peel to smooth out any remaining wrinkles, skin checking, or blemishing and to match up the skin to the age range of the new contours.

One adamant rule after a face peel is that the patient is allowed absolutely no sun bathing for six months. The general professional opinion is that *any* skin is better off without sun-bathing anyway.

This may change the long-standing unwritten rule of the Beautiful Jet Setters that sun-baked skin and sun-streaked hair are the only way to look. Or it may not.

110

They can afford to have a face peel every year, and a number of them do. And although a face peel can be repeated in 8 to 12 weeks if the initial peel is not wholly satisfactory, I do not approve of subjecting the skin and underlying tissues, as well as the entire organism to the effects of the acid solution even as often as every year.

The emergence of this "secret" youth weapon from the realm of the wealthy and the professional to a now "open secret" of the plastic surgeon's office has brought with it some fringe benefits as well.

Like all *sub rosa* items, the cost, which could have been, and generally was, astronomical with the little ladies of the secret formulas, is now considerably less in your plastic surgeon's office, in medical hands.

The status of the face peel has changed so radically that now there are medical papers on it coming out of Florida. In 1966, in their paper "An Endorsement of Facial Chemo-Surgery," published in the British Journal of Plastic Surgeons, John H. F. Batstone and D. Ralph Millard, Jr., M. D., of the University of Miami School of Medicine, state:

"Surgeons interested in results can no longer dismiss it [the acid face peel] as recondite and unsavoury. Its striking efficacy should not be dimmed because there is no knife in the kit, or because it has long been mediated by lay beauticians."

Dr. Perry A. Sperber, of Daytona Beach, in another medical paper, writes:

"The new technique—chemosurgery—which is really chemical plastic surgery, can reach all desired areas of the face, thus avoiding contrasts in shades and hues between treated and untreated areas." (This is meant in contrast to dermabrasion, or planing, another process which removes the outer layer of skin mechanically by use of a rotary brush.)

If chemical surgery is not a replacement for plastic surgery, it is still a means of accomplishing much without surgery. The result can sometimes be like a movie—the calendar pages flipping backward to denote the regression of time.

Who gets peeled? It can be a teenager suffering from acne or a young woman who was left with scarring as a result of acne or chicken pox.

It can be a woman in her eighties—it's not uncommon—who wants to remove the etched map of the years, or a woman in her thirties who may want to "freshen up" her skin checking, light wrinkling and the ravages of sun-tanning, or get rid of some permanent blotching or blemishing.

The art of peeling can, in fact, progress from the face and hands to the shoulders and upper chest right down to the cleavage.

Patients have been known to pay as high as $10,000 for "the works." Again, plastic surgery says that it is dangerous to do such wide areas at the same time because of the amount of phenol absorbed by the system.

There is actually no way of knowing how much acid will penetrate and reach body organs. A medical knowledge of anatomy as well as of skin tissue is of extreme importance because of the real and very present danger of scarring or blotching from the effects of the acid as well. A chemical face lift should be done by hands no less qualified than those that do a surgical face lift.

The truth is that, reluctant as they were to give it medical sanction and status, the one technique plastic surgeons are still reluctant to perform is chemosurgery.

But there is a need for it in our youth-minded society—and a need creates a demand that must be answered. Even the rather tricky art of creating a new skin becomes more commonplace and a general part of the plastic surgeon's daily bookings.

There is no secret made of the fact that the skin peel is painful for the first few hours, and medication cannot entirely obviate it. One woman equated it with going through the flames of hell. Yet have I ever heard a patient, on viewing the results, say she would never go through it again? I have not. On the contrary. Even the ever-present uncertainty of results is overcome by the optimism and hope of the human spirit.

Even after the worst period, in the first two or three days, I see a difference in the very step of a patient returning to the office to

112

have the tape mask removed. By the time she is applying the thymol iodide powder, you can't tell what her face looks like, but the lift of her spirit shows in every movement of her body.

The wealthy dowager who gets together a group of friends at her Palm Beach estate—and flies in her favorite plastic surgeon to give them all face peels—is fading out of the picture along with the very word "dowager."

The secrecy is passing, and with it, the legendary dangers. It is no longer a situation of "your hacienda or mine?" (whether the patient came to the face peeler or vice versa.)

Instead of a "wrinkle farm," there is the plastic surgeon's office, where you can have a chemical face lift in the hour and a half it takes, and go home. Providing, of course, there is someone along to take you home, and to care for you when you get there.

Being an "outpatient" may not be as luxurious as flying your surgeon into your Palm Beach villa or even as a stay at a clinic in Rome or Switzerland. But it is a great deal more practical—in time, convenience and cost.

It is no longer the in-thing of the rich and famous to schedule a face peel as needed, or the dangerous thing in the hands of the unqualified, with both factors going together all too often.

It's also safe to say that skin is in—and thinking about it is no longer confined to the rarefied world of professionally beautiful and vital people.

The fun-fashion fakery that came in with the latter half of the 60s is only a put-on for the real. It doesn't really work otherwise.

And as much as anything, the skin—by itself or under that frank or even interestingly weird makeup—has got to be for real.

Even plastic surgery has caught up with that!

CHAPTER 10

Implants: Chins to Cheekbones

IT is not only possible, it is commonly accepted procedure, to put small, permanent silicone inserts under the cheekbones to give them and the face a new definition.

It can't be said for certain, but this technique was probably developed for all the round-faced, apple-cheeked girls who yearn for glamorous hollows and seek out plastic surgeons to see if they can't get them!

Chins can be augmented with implants or bone grafts. The result is cosmetic, but it is really reconstructive surgery. The correction of chins and jaws, which falls into as many categories as there are kinds of faces, actually comes under the category of rebuilding faces, while the reshaping of ears can be considered the annex.

Having the ears pinned back is one of the simplest and most common of plastic surgery operations.

Protruding ears are considered a congenital anomaly. During the third month of gestation, the auricle has already protruded from the side of the head, and by the sixth month the ear is fully formed on the embryo.

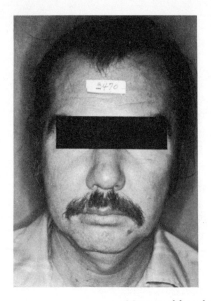 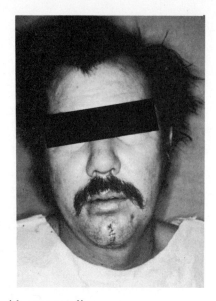

39-year-old male with very receding chin and little neck. Had chin enlargement and contouring of neck in one procedure. Result immediately post-operative.

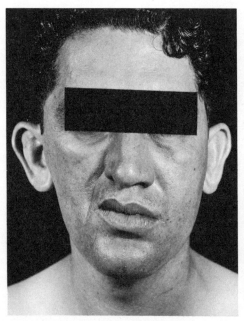 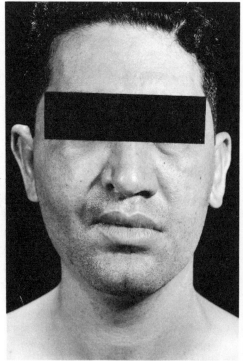

38-year-old man who had congenital hemiatrophy (loss) of the right side of his face and "dumbo ears." Had a silicone insert in his face and repair of ears.

The ear is the one feature on the child that is really father of the man, to quote Wordsworth out of context. By the age of five it is about ninety percent developed, and leaves little doubt as to what kind of ear the owner was lucky or unlucky enough to have inherited.

There is no "outgrowing" an asymmetrical ear, although the

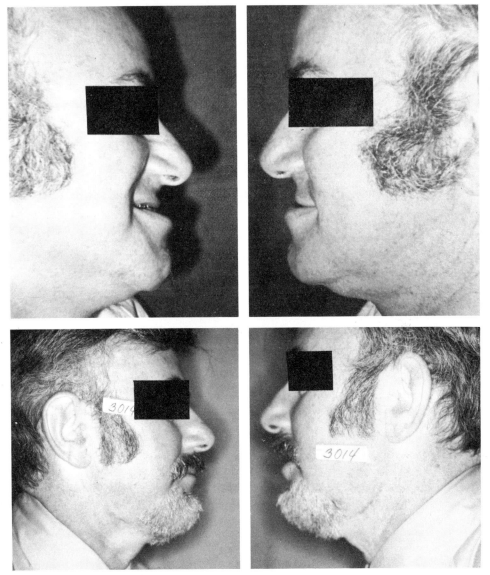

40-year-old man who had jaw set back. Result at six months.

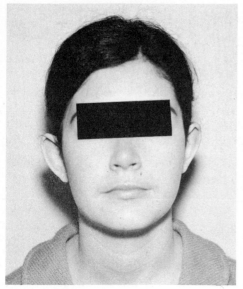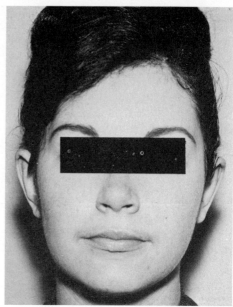

19-year-old female had otoplasty.
Result after one year.

hopeful outlook is that as the face gets larger the ear may become less prominent.

In this area, the males have had it over the females in having their ears pinned back. The face of a short-haired male appears even more bare and defenseless when framed by a pair of cup handle ears. With girls, the hair is supposed to hide those appendages on the side of the head. But with hair length a matter of variation, the statistics may change.

I had plenty of opportunity to observe such hereditary factors while stationed at the USAF Hospital at Wright-Patterson Air Force Base as chief of plastic surgery.

Just how hereditary ears are was pointed up by a case where the wife of an Air Force man brought in their two sons, ages five and six, to have their decidedly protuberant ears "fixed." The mother told me the other kids had taken to calling them Dumbo One and Dumbo Two. I took one look at *her* and asked, "Well, how about your own ears?" A beatific smile spread over her features as she said diffidently, "Well, doctor, if it is not too much trouble."

There are all kinds of variations of malformed ears, from the ones that stick out of, to the ones that stick to, the scalp (having never disassociated themselves), to cat's ears that flop over at the top, and other such oddities.

Sometimes the over-all height and width of the ear is in good proportion to the size and shape of the head, but the ear is not set right. The otoplasty, or ear operation, usually consists of re-modeling the ear cartilage and then resetting the ear in the proper position on the head. There are no visible scars, since the suturing is done in the crease behind the ear. Naturally, since it is entirely external, the reconstruction of the ear has no bearing or effect on the hearing.

The operation usually takes an hour and is very successfully done under a local anesthetic. There is little pain, and the bandage usually comes off within 5 days. There is no disturbance of the hair, since a surgical stockinette is worn over the head during the operation.

To avoid any possibility of injury, I usually have the patient wear a small bandage while sleeping for perhaps a few weeks. Ear muffs are a very handy way of protecting the ears while in bed during this time, without the necessity for bandaging.

Not everyone is part of an Air Force family with access to plastic surgery, courtesy of the government. But a woman who brought her two boys in had the right idea about *when* to have ears corrected. Before school is the ideal time, for two reasons.

Any corrective surgery that can be done early is best done then. The amount of reaction is minimal in a child, and he will not have to endure the taunts of his contemporaries at school about his too-obvious ears.

Parents who have passed on such ears to their children and have not had their own corrected will understand this without having it pointed out to them.

The chin and jaw are considered really intricate areas, although in reality the operations can be relatively simple.

It is still part of our mental conditioning that although re-doing the nose is accepted, tampering with the chin means something else again.

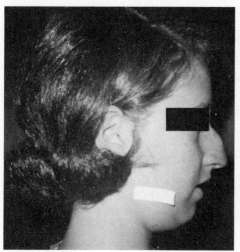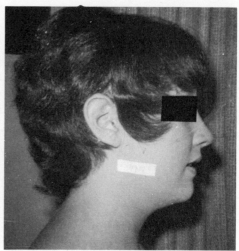

18-year-old female had rhinoplasty
and chin augmentation.

There was the 31-year-old Air Force pilot who had fractured his nose in 1954 while playing basketball. When I got him at the Wright-Patterson Air Force Base Hospital in 1965, he had a history of increased difficulty in breathing during those eleven years. Aside from the deformity of the fracture, a dorsal hump with off-center deviation to the left of the nose itself, the breathing passage of the left nostril was almost continuously closed. A septiplasty corrected the breathing, and the rhinoplasty straightened what had been a slightly humped nose (from the accident) with a natural unattractive droop to the tip.

The plain fact was that the pilot had the sort of "rabbit" profile that shows a droopy nose over a receding chin. The straightening of the nose brought the size of the chin into better conformity; a slight build-up of the chin would now bring his face into a pleasing symmetry.

It wasn't a question of changing a rugged male look, which can be attractive without being handsome. Some asymmetrical features have their own charm, giving a face an appealing individuality. Others are somehow just not right. I suggested the chin operation as an adjunct to the work on his nose, but he refused.

It was all right to have his nose fixed so he could breathe, with

120

the considerable outer improvement as a sort of dividend. But somehow the idea of re-doing his chin—which his own eyes could tell him would be an improvement—offended his idea of maleness.

The chin has so much to do with the final effect of the face that usually it is relatively simple to effect a startling change.

The lack of chin somehow gives an impression of something lacking in the person, something ineffectual. Too much chin has the opposite effect, giving an appearance of pugnaciousness. Both are equally unappealing. Sometimes an otherwise good chin just gets lost in fat. (This can usually be taken care of with the face lift.)

Double chins *can* be eliminated by themselves, however, if the patient needs no other surgery. The turkey wattle is a different matter, with the loose, hanging skin under the chin extending into the neck. By the time a person reaches the stage of a turkey wattle neck, further correction of the face is called for if the final result is to be satisfactory.

Resculpting the chin can be as simple as making an incision under the chin muscle and inserting an implant of silicone or

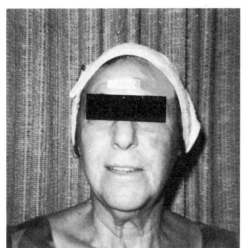 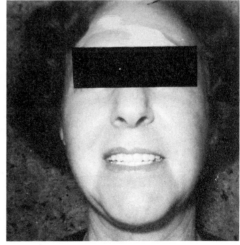

72-year-old lady who had chemical
face peel and repair of turkey neck.

121

HOW TO WIN IN THE YOUTH GAME

teflon. The incision can go through the mouth in the buccal sulcus mucosa and generally fades away of itself in about six months.

This can be done—I *prefer* it done—under a local anesthetic. It takes less than half an hour, and after two weeks the change is permanent: the kind of chin the face should have had in the first place if nature hadn't goofed.

There are much more intricate chin corrections, depending on the teeth, the jaw, the bite, even the kind of bone the patient has. Sometimes the chin operation will correct the occlusion, or bite, with teeth being realigned at the same time by some ancillary dental work.

Sometimes even additional bone will be required in reshaping a chin. It can come from the bone banks available for this purpose or from the patient's own hip. And in some cases correction of both the chin *and* jaw are done at the same time. In this case, usually too much jaw goes with too large a chin, which can make for various effects from the commonly titled protruding or "lantern" jaw to an anthropoid look to a simply unattractive heavy lower face (in the case of women, especially). These conditions, like ears, are usually hereditary and run in families.

Some of the jaw operations, usually entailing surgery from inside the mouth and cutting away excess bone, may require having the jaws wired for as long as two months.

Correcting protruding or otherwise malformed jaws and under- or over-sized chins is often far from being a matter of vanity or aesthetics.

Aside from the appearance, there is often malocclusion, causing the wearing away of teeth and inability to chew properly. To add to that, the position of the lips is determined by the formation of the chin-jaw line. A correction of *it* can affect the looks of the mouth, although it has not been touched. Sometimes several wisdom teeth on either side may have to be extracted to get the optimum results.

Since the chin-jawline is hereditary, it is again obvious that the child is not going to outgrow such malformations. But unlike the ears, which are eighty percent formed by the age of five or even

122

before that, the chin, like the nose, doesn't stop growing before age eighteen.

There are some malformations that should not wait until growth has stopped, since they can cause further difficulty with muscle and tissue. The thinking now is that the chin correction can be done successfully on quite young children, influencing proper development of jaw and teeth.

Because of the effects of a badly receding chin—from an improper bite to an insulted psyche—it is best to have the correction done at the earliest time the surgeon deems advisable.

Such reconstruction is not always done to correct a nature who was not at her best (and we do see examples every day that nature can be downright imperfect), but just as frequently, the need is accidental. As an example, there was a 22-year-old boy brought in from a freeway crash with bone fractures of the mandibles. Succinctly, the damage could be described as broken jaws, both of them. To complicate the case, his dental arch had to be put back in place and the teeth realigned in proper relationship.

That's a lot harder than improving on some of the unnatural creations of nature.

Reconstruction of the lower face is done for many reasons and sometimes even with extra advantages. I like the reaction of the patient who, although her mouth had not been touched while she was getting a new chin, smiled, "I am more kissable now."

CHAPTER 11

Quick Cosmetic Surgery:
Silicone to Sanding

IF silicone were really as bad as it is being bad-mouthed, women would be walking around with weights in the bottoms of their breasts.

It's not so bad, but it's not so good either. There is an uncertainty factor. It is definitely true that silicone does travel in the body and that there is no way to control it. It has caused some weird reactions, even some sad jokes, based on the truth that there are some women whose silicone injections have traveled to the bottom of their breasts.

The further consideration about silicone is more pragmatic. Liquid silicone injection is not to be confused with solid silicone implants.

The Food and Drug Administration has had liquid silicone injection under study since around 1965. Its status has never been absolutely clear, but it has been going through various steps, with the banning of it at first for breast use, but not for face, hands and other parts of the body.

125

However, since the FDA has confiscated all known supplies of liquid silicone, it can be presumed that its use is illegal. Any silicone procurable would not be from Dow Corning, which makes the medical silicone, and therefore would be of a dubious source and quality in itself.

Yet articles on cosmetic surgery do still include silicone injection. The fact is that it is being used to pump out both wrinkles and hollows in both face and hands.

The limbo status of liquid silicone is rather a pity. It was first discovered in Japan as a means of plumping out withered legs in polio patients. But it's up to the FDA to have the final word.

The silicone needle is one of the quick cosmetic surgicals you can't have. But there are others you can have.

The electric needle can get rid of so many bothersome surface developments in such short order that it's a mystery why people walk around wishing they could get rid of those broken red capillaries, yet don't do anything about the condition. Or, worse, those age spots that decorate the hands and other parts of the body.

Broken blood vessels (spider nevi) that make those tiny red lines on the nose, and the liver spots can be touched out with the needle. The charge of electricity that goes from the needle to the offending broken red vein makes the walls of the vein or capillary stick together so no blood comes through any more. Ergo, you don't see the red.

One very fair-skinned actress got too much sun one summer and developed some broken capillaries on her chest. She wore high necked clothes until she found what a minor matter it was to remove them.

The removal of liver spots produces scabs, which take about a week to disappear. There is no anesthetic needed, and the job is done generally in a matter of minutes. But, of course, it depends on how much of a job there is to do. A large nest of *telangiectasias* on nose or cheek or legs may take a number of visits, while a few can be obliterated by a touch of the needle.

Leg veins—red and blue traceries—take longer because they're

126

larger. If they're complicated, the treatment may be protracted, but, yes, they can be removed.

Moles and warts lend themselves to chemical removal or cryosurgery (freezing) or to removal in most cases by the needle.

Warts, particularly, should have attention as soon as they appear. Warts are caused by a virus (which is why sometimes they go away by themselves—but don't depend on it). They are harmless in themselves, but they are infectious to the one who has the wart, so he can keep infecting himself and grow new ones. If a wart is neglected too long, its removal can leave a scar.

Dermabrasion is also one of the quicker marvels. Lately it seems to have given over to chemical peeling, but it can still have a variety of uses in eliminating some undesirable factors.

As against skin peeling, done with chemicals, dermabrasion (skin planing) is done with a tiny electric brush. It *is* somewhat akin to planing wood. If you go too deep the wood is uneven. If you go too deep with dermabrasion you get scarring.

That's no reason not to consider it, if you put yourself into competent hands. There's every reason to consider it, when those upper lip wrinkles can be removed or minimized in the space of ten minutes. It can be done with a local anesthetic, or the skin can be frozen with a spray of air and chemical.

Dermabrasion can lessen a multitude of surface sins: from acne to freckles and nowadays even tattoos. And wrinkles can be planed down, too.

As to how successfully it can work for you and how much can be done, only your plastic surgeon can tell you definitely. But it's one more way *not* to have to live with the annoying, the embarrassing and the unlovely.

127

CHAPTER 12

The Emerging Male
Has Hair on His Head

IN the youth sweepstakes, men have it over women. They are not only physically designed to look better longer, but their lives are also designed for a minimal fraction of daily upkeep compared to a woman's.

It may be men who get the heart attacks, but did you ever hear a man say, "I washed my hair and I can't do a thing with it?" He's apt to reply, as I heard one say to his wife, "At least you have hair."

Men, as a matter of course, concentrate on the natural while a woman's whole psychology is to depend on artifice. Well, not really artifice. Enhancement.

Today's Organization Man is apt to be two people. On the job he still isn't too far out for the Establishment, even if he is out of the old buttoned-down Madison Avenue grey flannel uniform and into something a little easier.

Away from the job, though, he's apt to be the company swinger. He not only puts more hair on his head than the office would stand for, he might add a mustache to longer sideburns. He can even stick on a chest muff to make him look—and feel?—more masculine. Even for the humdrum workday, he uses hair spray and a touch of cologne.

The revolution leading to all this started with men wearing beads over their hippy tunics or Nehru jackets.

And how much they got caught in the same trap as women's fashion showed when the Nehru went as dead as the dodo bird in a few months. There are still untold thousands of Nehrus, those that haven't been turned over to the gardener or handyman or the Goodwill, hanging in the backs of closets, mute symbols of the masculine sartorial liberation.

The real meaning of the Male Revolution *was* that a man's article of apparel could go out of style as whimsically as a woman's.

The Male Revolution it is. And the only question about it, men, is: What took you so long? For over 150 years, we forgot that in nature it is the *male* peacock that opens that fantastic fan behind him while the female is a drab little hen; it is the lion who sports the handsome ruff around his neck while the lioness looks bare and even scrawny by comparison; that in nature it is the male who sports the plumage.

And we have lost track of the fact that the human male has through history sported some fancy plumage of his own. Don't just look at Liberace, look at some of the costumes assembled by the courtiers at the court of the Louis's.

Why, our own present day swinger hasn't yet dared put on anything as colorful as the wig and knee breeches, with buckled shoes, worn by our own George Washington.

Men simply went into a decline of drabness with the industrial revolution. Although once they started, they came back pretty fast, but it has still been step by step.

The idea of *men* wearing beads was pretty incredible, and when they got so common as to become outré, the next "you can't be serious" item was handbags.

The fashion world has come up with some quite handsome shoulder bags to be carried by men—real men—that, for all their ease of handling, seem no more anachronistic than an attaché case. For that matter, they seem to be an evolvement of the standard attaché case.

Naturally, the next step was midi skirts for men. Hollywood types like Frank Sinatra, Peter Fonda, Ross Hunter, and Roger Vadim—plus *everybody*—took on an exotic, dashing look in the leisure wear department.

If those short tutus worn by those famous Greek Ladies from Hell in battle make them look like male ballet dancers and kilts make Scotsmen look handsomer, the midi skirt managed to make the male jet set type look as if he were ready for a karate lesson. And by now, there is nothing strange about it at all.

What took the male so long to recapture his lost plumage? For one thing, when he went into his penguin era, we had all acquired the conditioning that men were men and women were women and never the twain would meet—in material accoutrements.

What with men getting into skirts, even if only for the casual life, and women already wearing pants, we went through phases of labelling, as if biology had had its own revolution, too. Men were being trans-sexed; women, especially the women libbers, were being de-sexed. And under the whole tent, there was the ultimate threat of unisex.

What it all amounted to was more of a de-polarization than a de-sexing or un-sexing. If a woman can wear pants, why *can't* a man wear a skirt? In the Chinese culture that *was* the order. The lava-lavas from which our own men got their own natty leisure skirts are worn by those fierce, muscled, fighting South Sea Islanders.

De-polarization is simply an emergence of long suppressed good sense—on both sides. Body clothes, garments made to the requirements of a living, moving body, don't have *any* sexual label. Knits, formerly feminine to the nth power, are now a standard part of male clothes that move with freedom; but they are knits that look woven, and cut into traditional suits and classic jackets.

But when anything happens too fast, people are wont to flee back into something secure. We have even gone through a post-

131

revolution push to send peacocks back to the nest—where things can get hennishly dull and drab. The counterrevolution had about as much validity as (remember?) when, following the London clothing quake that brought on the new age, they were going around saying, "Mod is dead." Whatever "they" meant!

It may take getting used to, in having something you never had before. But getting used to isn't giving up!

Can you imagine a man's using his wife's face cream a few short years ago? Even the thought wouldn't have occurred to him. Today he's putting on *her* moisturizer at night, and not sneaking it either.

Men didn't really miss being shut out of the world of strictly feminine fripperies. A room full of women in the same dresses would have to look like a stage production number, but a room full of men in the same dark suits has an appealingly masculine aura.

The fact is that men look better than women. As is, that is. Which one do you think would be more at ease with himself or herself if found in that romantic situation of being cast away on a desert island?

Cartoons always picture such castaways with the man looking like a refugee from skid row and a ragtag stubble on his face, while the woman always manages to look like a model of Al Capp's sexy Daisy Mae.

Actually, if you stop to think about it—and who hasn't, at one time or other?—if they'd been marooned long enough, the man would probably be looking appealingly raffish with a full beard, while the lady would most probably look as if she would rather be invisible until she could get back to some civilized grooming.

The male, in his superiority, has been wily enough to become accepted for what he is by nature. The female has built up a whole concept of herself that *improves* on nature. Therein lies her whole snare and delusion.

Of course, men aren't prettier than women. But they do *look* better than women not only in the acceptance of their utter maleness, but by their natural equipment.

132

Men don't have as much fat under their skin as women; they have more muscle. That keeps them firmer than women longer, even if the fat that women have keeps them warmer and softer.

A man, by virtue of needing to use that muscle, will be more apt to work out regularly in a gym, as a matter of course, which *keeps* him fit. Give a man a good game of handball, or a workout at the gym, followed by a massage, and he can come out looking fit, fresh of skin and bright of eye.

It's not quite the same as a woman spending the afternoon at a beauty salon, is it?

But now we're getting to co-ed gyms, as a later development. If *he's* invading what was formerly her domain, then she's learning that fat goes to flab if it's not exercised. That's the kind of unisex that works!

We are coming to realize the formerly unthinkable; that in the proper hormonal balance, no man is *all* male or any woman *all* female. Each has a little of the other's hormone in his makeup. As with any rigid distinctions, eventually there must be some give and take in both directions. Once we are past the usual puzzlements and adjustments, to the truth revealed, in the long run things become easier and freer all the way around.

Robert Burns said "A man's a man for a' that," and so he is. He's just getting out of his suit of armor to show that he's human, not superhuman. It used to be that man was supposed to disdain the artifices of women; now he's not only taking advantage of them, he's running to catch up.

As for his superior musculature, he's come to realize that he's only human in that respect, too, and that it doesn't hold up forever.

To get down to cases, plastic surgery in the masculine department used to be had almost exclusively by men in the theatre, TV or movies, who had to keep up their looks.

Even so, a full face lift for a man was a rarity, mainly because it was considered that his hair was too short to hide the scar at the back of his neck.

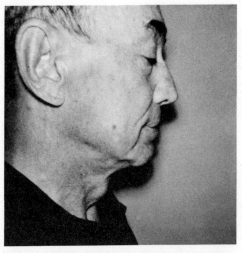

67-year-old male who underwent rhytidectomy and blepharoplasty. Result after one year.

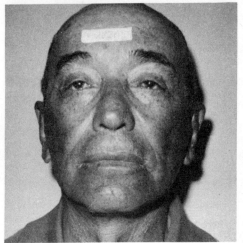

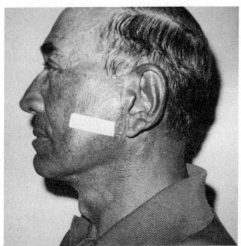

Today, fifteen to twenty percent of all *full* face lifts are performed on men. Bankers, lawyers, executives who need to keep up their appearance, are matched by men who just *want* to—and visit the plastic surgeon. There no longer has to be any reason other than just wanting to look better and more fit.

Men are running the full gamut of plastic surgery performed for women—from a *blepharoplasty* to remove those bags under the eyes, and incidentally, to get a more wide-awake look—to having the skin tautened on a "chicken neck," to having a skin peel to wipe off the erosion of years and those hard-to-take pressurized board meetings.

Men have become so much a part of the usual in plastic surgery, that one recent Friday night when my nurse brought in the schedule of the following week's operations, I looked at it and commented with surprise, "Mostly women? Not many men."

Perhaps the most remarkable—no, it really is the most remarkable—recent triumph of man over his outward appearance

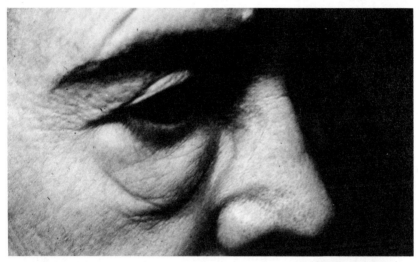

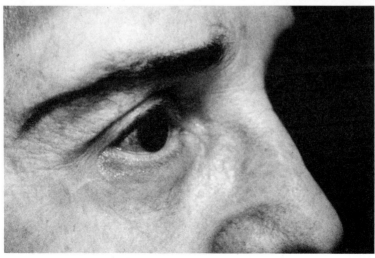

70-year-old man had repair of upper and lower eyelids. Result after three weeks.

has been in the area that easily plagued him the most and seemed the most hopeless. Burlesque is gone, and now it seems that the "baldhead row" that was its mainstay is on the way to becoming a thing of the past as well. Baldheaded men may become an extinct species, and soon. In fact, they are *now* becoming extinct, as fast as they can get their hair transplants.

After all the years of searching for an inward panacea, with all the grasping at straw hopes of bringing back lost hair by means of hormones or proteins, it is now possible to grow hair again. Real hair.

Science has finally become satisfied that, up to the present, there is no known internal route to cure baldness, that nothing of that kind will really bring back lost hair.

Hair is a generic time table, dependent on heredity. When it's gone, it's gone. Why does hair fall out? Why does it fall out from the top—in what is called the classic male-pattern baldness—and why do otherwise bald men have hair on the back and sides of their heads?

There is no answer except that, maybe, it was designed to grow that way until hair implants were discovered by plastic surgery.

Hair implants are simply taking the hair from where it *does* grow—and implanting it permanently where it no longer grows. Hair transplants are nothing more than compatible skin grafts. They're the same as skin grafting on a burn.

Just as the composition of the graft must be compatible with all the natural layers of skin being replaced, the fat, tissue and hair follicle must be consistent in the hair transplant. If you don't have the root, the hair will fall out. By putting the root in, you are planting real, honest-to-goodness, growing hair.

There are various ways to do hair transplants or implants—the terms are interchangeable because you are taking hair from area and planting it on another. If you've got that Nero fringe, you've got hair!

The most common method of transplant is the punch, where little holes are dug in the scalp to receive the new hair plugs. In a way, it's like planting your garden.

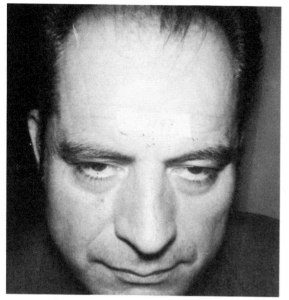
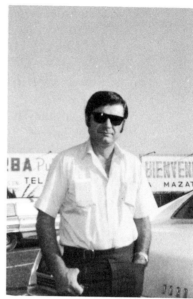

40-year-old man who has undergone 400 hair implants over a two-
year-period. Result after two years.

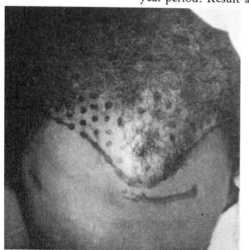
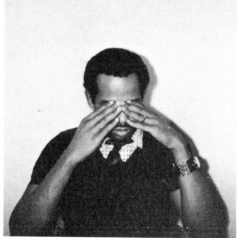

38-year-old man who had 300 hair
plugs. Result at one year.

Yes, there is some bleeding, and the noise beating on your brains is something like a woodpecker at work on his tree, if you're not in the "twilight zone." It may be done under a local anesthetic, and while some patients can't take too much of it at a time, others don't seem to mind at all. (I had mine awake and didn't like it.)

How long does it take? It depends on how much hair you need—or want—to replace, how often you can come in for a session, and other such personal factors.

There is the millionaire playboy who came up from Miami, checked into a hotel, checked in with me and said, "Just tell me how long I have to stay, Doc."

He had called me first from Miami to say that he had had an implant that wasn't satisfactory and wanted me to see if anything could be done. He had had about 300 plugs, of which perhaps fifty actually took. Too much had been done too soon to be supported by the blood supply. There must be time to establish the new circulation by keeping the blood flowing, so that each session prepares the scalp for the next, with each succeeding implant helping the other.

The hair can be transplanted in plugs, or it can be done in strips, perhaps four inches long and an eighth of an inch wide, or in combination.

This man's hair was still thinning, so I gave him a new hairline with strips and inserted plugs behind that, so that all the hair would comb in together. We spaced the time out so that the whole process took 18 days.

A big session would be 80 to 120 plugs, and from 500 to 1000 may be needed. A short session, perhaps at the end of the day, might be as few as 10 plugs. (I do not understand these quoted "twice a day" visits. The rest of the procedure aside, how can anyone want a local anesthetic twice a day?) Some people just make appointments as they would at a dentist—until the work is accomplished.

What do you do while the implant is "taking?" No, it isn't actually "instant" hair. The new follicle goes into shock, and the hair itself generally falls out. You have to wait for it to come up again, like anything else that is planted.

There has to be a scaling off of the scab from the implant, and after that, you won't see anything for three weeks to three months. Of course, you'll be doing a lot of looking in the mirror at your scalp in the interim.

The first thing you will see is fuzz—an astonishing beautiful sight to the spirit. The fuzz turns into real, growing hair. And it will continue to grow, if you have had the proper medical procedure and care, as long as the site from which it was taken doesn't go bald. Usually, that Nero's fringe that always remains at the sides and back, which is the donor site, stays with the wearer for life.

It would seem that the hair doesn't know it was transplanted, but acts as if it were still growing from the home site it was taken from. That's an anomaly—or perhaps a fact of nature—that we can't exactly explain, but that's the way it is.

What does one do while this process is taking place? Fortunately, implanting real hair has been paced by the manufacture of hair that doesn't grow but that you put on. A man can cover what is going on with a fake hair piece that is a facsimile of what will soon be for real. Some men, planning well ahead, start wearing that put-on hair *before* the implanting starts, so they and people who see them in their daily life get used to it.

Women, who wear wigs as a matter of course anyway, really don't have a problem. They just wear a wig during the period they are getting back some real hair. And if you don't think *women* need hair implants, you should come to my office and learn about *that*! It used to be considered that women just didn't lose their hair—hence, I think, the term, *male*-pattern baldness.

I don't know if with women baldness was a better kept secret, because of their longer hair, but I do know that women lose their hair too. Everybody loses some hair to age, when it just naturally gets thinner. But women of all ages—many of them in their thirties—often have distressing bald spots under that hairdo or hairpiece.

The fashion of frankly fake hair has been a boon to more women than you might imagine. Some of them have said to me, "What would I ever do without it?" Nevertheless, although almost every woman now has her collection of hair-pieces and wigs openly displayed, it doesn't make up for the real thing. Ergo, hair transplants are no longer exclusively a man's domain or necessity.

The way hair grows is perhaps more idiosyncratic than any other area in which plastic surgery is involved. That is why the early days of this new technique—which were no more than a few years ago—did see some pretty odd results, at high cost.

The hairline, the direction the hair grows, the placing of the plugs, are all an integral part of a successful hair implant. Today, it is part of the plastic surgery technique, with the time consumed and the cost more in keeping with what they should be.

Hair implants have saved the careers of many a TV actor and commentator. In fact, hair is so important when you're in front of a camera that hair implanting has become a fact of life with entertainment figures.

Whereas just a few years ago they got some pretty weird results at times—there is one particularly famous name among them who never has gotten his to look right—today they will come in at random to have a few new plugs adroitly placed.

One such character, when called by a friend and asked what he was doing, answered, "Standing here cursing and watching my hair fall out." Today, that head in front of the camera isn't getting less hair, it's growing more and more luxuriant.

Like all the rest of our advantages that we have come to live by, having hair is no longer a condition confined to entertainment figures or lucky people.

In fact, men don't care a fig about being considered virile because they're bald.

They'd rather have hair.

CHAPTER 13

Food and How to Stay Away From It

His food was glory, which was poison
to his mind and peril to his body.

Sir Henry Taylor

OTTO PREMINGER talking:
 "I am on a diet."
 "What kind of a diet?"
 "I don't eat."
Who could have expressed it better than Otto? Not even the
greatest nutritionist extant. Of *all* the diets—from nutty to nutri-
tional—that have been hopefully started, science itself has at last
come to the conclusion that the best diet of all is the no-food diet.

The combination of mother (and not necessarily the Jewish
mother) stuffing food into the child and the emphasis of nutri-
tional findings (that we need sixty grams of this and 110 milli-
grams of that each day or we will in some way disintegrate) has
been too much.

There is a lingering unease in the mind about *not* eating. But it
is now a known fact of life that a little fasting doesn't hurt. For
those with the fortitude to fast, they find it does a wonder-
working amount of good. Those prophets who went into the

wilderness and fasted knew what it was all about. It not only clears the skin and lightens the body—it gives the mind a soaring clarity that is a great experience in itself.

Food, of course, is necessary as fuel for the human machine. The only trouble is that we use a richer mixture than we need. When you do that with your car, you get exhaust fumes. When you do it with your body, you get—well, see the quote from old Sir Henry Taylor, the nineteenth century forerunner of Otto Preminger.

Evidently, Sir Henry wasn't just talking, because he managed to live from 1800-1886, not a bad life span, even for today.

The whole trouble with eating is that, aside from its function to fuel the body so it can run, it also satisfies some psychological and emotional hungers. To make it worse, eating is part of our socially active civilization. Not to speak of how good chocolate cake tastes.

So the fact is that many of us eat far more than we actually need, with distressing results. And we eat without thinking. To amend the old cliché that inside every fat man there is a thin man struggling to get out—he isn't struggling hard enough.

But the meaning sums up the whole struggle. The person who is eating actually *is* two people: the one who is eating for eating's sake is not caring about what happens to the body of the other one, who says of the first one, "I don't *like* her." (Or him.)

People are prone to think of themselves as *me*—someone who lives inside of them. What they don't realize is that *me* is created to a large extent by how they look and feel.

The amount of food we require, as against the amount we want and what it does to us, is out of whack. Just think of your stomach as an incinerator, consuming that stuff coming into it and sending it out through the various, awesomely marvelous machinations of the body into your cells, tissue, skin, blood and brain. Are you throwing garbage into it? Because that's what excess food becomes.

Once you have managed to imprint this in indelible red ink on your mind, the idea of overeating may even become repulsive to you. Which, in actuality, it is. It can even put that chocolate cake in its proper category.

If you have trouble staying away from the refrigerator, and it's a very common disease, there are numerous reminder slogans as a cure to tack up on that piece of kitchen furniture. Have you tried: *Do I Want To Be Repulsive?*

If you *are* going to overfuel yourself—with all the resultant physical smog from the too high food octane—at least know yourself well enough to know *why* you are doing it. There's no remedy for anything until you understand the reason.

The stomach, too, learns habits and becomes conditioned to them. *Especially* the stomach! Overeating may be just a bad, undisciplined habit you learned in childhood, when food was good for you, a panacea for hurts, a reward. Even today, a TV commercial pretends that all the little frustrations of life can be helped by a piece of a particular brand of frozen cake. Amusing, but a naughty come-on.

The more you put into your stomach, the more it becomes accustomed to. It wants to fill up to the size it has been stretched to. That's why the first stages of the diet are so tough. The stomach is unsatisfied and, therefore, uncomfortable, because you're not treating it in the style it has become accustomed to. You now have to *reverse* the process, so that it shrinks to a smaller capacity—and you and it become *more* comfortable.

There are any number of reasons why people crave food satisfaction, aside from just having learned from doting mothers to overeat.

Food *is* love, a fact established at the very onset of life when mother nurses (or feeds) her child—and a gut feeling that can cause mischief all through the rest of life. Food can make up for frustration, rejection, failure, a lousy sex life—all the human inadequacies we have to cope with.

So when you go on that uncontrollable eating binge, at least use your brain along with your mouth to realize why. If you *have* to go ahead, anyway, go ahead. But if you have conditioned yourself to looking inward and realizing *why,* reason may in time triumph over emotion and you might *stop*!

Think about why, when and how you are overeating. *Keep* thinking about it, even *while* you are gorging uncontrollably. No one thing works alone within the organism. Mind and body work together. Discipline begins with a consciousness of what you really want. When you really know that, discipline becomes a habit.

Fat is an equation. Too much food is what equals too much flesh. Do you really need it? Develop a taste for thinness that's stronger than your taste for unnecessary food.

If people can stop smoking—and I know a number who did just that: stop—they can stop overeating, as well. It is really a question of convincing *yourself* that you are not going to overeat because it is making less of a human being of you, while you are more of a human being than you should be (on the scale). Psychological reasons and motivations for overeating are all well and good, and you should understand yourself in relation to them.

A *motivation* for not overeating may be stashing those size 8 clothes in the closet until you fit them, or wanting to lose weight because you have found someone you care about, and that's when not having the body to live up to the occasion really matters. As Helen Gurley Brown put it in that deathless phrase, "The body is what you make love with."

I have even known people to take off weight easily when they're looking forward to taking a special trip or vacation—so they'll be able to enjoy it.

But in the long run, your appearance should be your own best motivation. And if you think enough of yourself, you won't need any other reason.

Vitality or grossness? It actually becomes as simple as that, because it is still true that what you are putting into your body is what it becomes. Let alone the skin flareup that comes after all that chocolate, the very excretions of the body change with the food you put into it.

And when you *know* you're indulging in sheer, simple sin instead of creating good firm muscle and healthy tissue and glowing skin, be aware that all those starches and sugars are not only robbing your body of their natural vitamins, they're going to flaccid fat.

In other words: Why am I creating a *me* with all sorts of stumbling blocks for the sake of this food I don't need? It may seem like a cold-turkey approach, but until you really see it that way, the truth is that you're going to backslide, no matter how many different diets you go on. And there you go, in trouble again. Because it's much harder to take off those pounds than to put them on.

Fat is a hangup, and this is the age of getting rid of your hangups if you don't want to live with them.

By the next century, if it's any consolation, the fat problem may have solved itself. Along with the giddy promise that nobody will be old and everybody will be beautiful, nobody will be fat, either.

Food will possibly already come with the fatmakers removed. The idea of being nourished by a pill alone has been put forth for a long time, but the human mechanism is so constructed that it just wouldn't like it.

So unless we change the human mechanism, or lose our pleasure in eating, we will go on ingesting food. But it will be a different food than we have ever had. We will know more about it, as well as much more about its relationship to the human mechanism. And obviously no one will overeat because we shall have a different mental conditioning toward food.

We can do some of all this for ourselves, today, can't we? There are already enough "fat savers" in foods sweetened without whole sugar, fat substitutes, starchless flours and the like.

We can eat the salmon with cucumbers instead of potato salad, which is not only less heavy but more gourmet. And lobster without the Newburg, or dripping it with butter (lemon is really better).

145

We can eat the shrimp without the cracker, thereby appreciating the shrimp more, the steak without the potato but with a fine green salad.

Instead of that cream-layered Napoleon for dessert, there is fruit canned in its natural juice, even without the need for artificial sweetening. When they started canning, the processors didn't use the fruit's natural juice, but made a heavy sugar syrup to sweeten it. Even that's improving, so we must be coming along.

You've heard all this before—about leaving off the potato swimming in butter and making it a green salad, instead—but have you heard it often enough to *do* it? The end result of caring about what you eat is that you learn to enjoy your food more, not less.

In fact, the way you eat depends on whether you are underweight or overweight. Scientists have found that thin people respond to *internal* cues of body chemistry (hunger) while fat people respond to *external* cues: seeing is wanting, whether hungry or not. This would seem to indicate that to get thin is to stay thin. We all know, alas, that is not the happy fact, once we fall off that diet we went on to *get* thin.

People suffer through many phony diets and eventually undo them, lapsing back to their neurotic drives! The only diet is a thinking diet, one that puts food in its proper place. In its proper place for *you*.

Anybody will lose weight on a diet of 1,000 calories a day. But they can't live on 1,000 calories a day indefinitely. That's the big consideration. Calories *are* important, of course. But food is too important to us to live by a calorie count. And even the calorie has to be considered in relationship to other factors.

Is the calorie carbohydrate or protein? That's going to make a large difference in what your body is going to do with it. A piece of candy, say 250 calories of carbohydrate, is looked on as "fattening." But if you eat that piece of candy on an empty stomach (suppositional, not advisory!) it is going to be digested easily and quickly. If you eat a large dinner and then eat a similar piece of candy, it is just going to lie there, because your enzymes won't function in the same way.

146

That, by the way, is clogging up the body plumbing. Someone once asked me, "If the body is supposed to renew itself every seven years, how come we don't see this happen?"

The answer is right there. What man has been doing to his outer environment in pollution, he has also been doing to his inner environment. The cells do renew themselves, but the environment we create for them is so unsatisfactory that their quality becomes equated to it.

It is part of the disease known as the aging process.

So calorie consciousness alone is hardly the answer to getting and staying fit. Not all foods react the same way in all people either. It is good to know the values of foods but even better to understand what they to do you—as you.

Everyone knows that there are some foods that put weight on quicker than others, and the calorie value may not be at much variance. Listen to what your body is telling you about your relationship to food. If peanuts make you fat, switch to birdseed (only if you are a bird, of course)!

It is even known that a variety of foods actually stimulates the appetite. The digestive enzymes just run amok; their overactivity causes you to want to go on eating.

From this fact comes the mono-diet, meaning one food. There are all kinds of *good* fast diets from mono to melon, or maybe mono-melon for three days.

There are lettuce diets (this is close to the starvation diet of no food) and something much more easy to take, the wine diet.

The wine diet is wine and one egg, wine and two eggs, a small steak and finish the bottle of wine. This is one diet that may get the dieter a little tipsy—but he won't be able to deny that he's happy.

There's nothing wrong with going on a fast diet to start you taking the pounds off. It's an encouragement to start with. It's what happens after that that counts. The permanent happening, that is. Otherwise, you'll be like all the other diet freaks, up and down the scale.

There's only one real solution to the problem. EAT LESS!

147

Don't give up food. Only the food you don't need. And don't want, you tell yourself. Don't tell yourself with clenched fists and screwed tight eyes and an intense "I am not going to do this, I am not going to do this," in exclamation points.

Something in human consciousness often operates in a perverse manner, so that when you tell yourself, "I am not going to do this," you end up doing it. When you are concentrating too intensely on one thing, you are going to do that thing.

I know someone who quit smoking one day, cold turkey. No tapering off, no rituals of any kind, she (yes, she) just quit.

She didn't do it by will power, or concentration or anything like it. She did it rather by *not* thinking about it. She didn't say "I won't smoke." Instead she said, "I won't smoke today." It's been three years, and she still hasn't let herself know she quit smoking. What she did was to leave herself the leeway of choice. Like, if she really wanted to smoke, she would. She hasn't wanted to.

She thinks she did something to hypnotize herself into not wanting to smoke, because she honestly didn't suffer at any time for want of a cigarette. I think that, in some way, she picked the right psychological way for herself. If she had told herself she *couldn't* smoke, instead of wouldn't, she'd have climbed the walls.

What makes this really worthwhile is that she is a writer who had been conditioned for years to typing with a cigarette in one hand. The repair man used to scream about the ashes that casually went down into her typewriter as she hit the carriage. What surprised her most of all is that she didn't miss that cigarette in her left hand as she typed away with the right and a couple of fingers of the left. She even forgot the cigarette should be there.

She didn't substitute anything for the cigarette consciously, although in her case it might have been the work itself. Writing requires such concentration that it automatically shuts out everything else. This same writer, who works with the radio on, finds herself listening to the news as it starts, but she soon turns back to the typewriter unconsciously.

One axiom for eating less *is* to substitute some other interest for it. Certainly, haven't there been days when you have been too busy to concentrate on food and found that you didn't need it after all?

Getting in a new groove *can* very well substitute for an interest in food. Women generally lose weight when they fall in love, have an affair, or want to impress somebody.

But it's better to do it the really satisfying, lasting way, *with* an interest in food, so that you are aware of what you are doing about it. It's not only the difference in gourmet or glutton. It's allowing yourself the luxury of being fit, with a body that feels good, not overstuffed, with a clear skin and an easy vitality.

Then you don't have to get ready for life. You are ready.

CHAPTER 14

Passion Shadows and
the Now and Future Woman

WOMAN, since Eve, seems to have known instinctively what modern psychologists are telling her today. That is that her outer environment has a way of finding itself inside, and becoming part of her inner environment.

Researchers and anthropologists have encountered this truism throughout history. A makeup kit found in a royal tomb at Ur in Babylonia. The knowledge that good old Cleopatra, still the symbol for the *femme fatale,* had available in her day such items as brow and lash and hair dyes, bleaches and powders and rouge, and *yes*, moisturizers, as well as wrinkle creams, freckle cream, sunburn lotion, depilatories and lubricants and cleansing creams.

To bring this concern with the outer environment up to date, Dr. Ernest Dichter, a motivational researcher, said on National Educational Television: "When a woman applies cream, there's a sort of feeling of something magic happening."

Doesn't sound like things have really changed that much, in some five thousand years? But they have! The uses of artifice have

151

been improved upon with the ages. It was the physician Galen, in the second century A.D., who first came up with today's basic formula for cold cream: oil, beeswax and water.

While some methods of beauty and rejuvenation used in the past may have been lost to us, we are coming up constantly with some diverting and varied ones of our own.

They can come from the sea, they can be animal, vegetable, fruit or mineral, embryo or cellular, or they can be concocted in a test tube from combinations.

Beauty is a $7 billion annual business in the United States, if you include beauty salons with the cosmetics and toiletries sold over the counter.

Magazines continuously print articles on the state of Beauty and the Female, running from the overextended ones that talk about miraculous cosmetic changes to those (sometimes written by men) who take a head-patting, there-there attitude about the whole big thing, with the implication that it's all $7 billion worth of hope and feathers. As to whether the whole thing is only a female indulgence, aided and abetted by the beautiful promises of persuasive advertising copywriters, I have only one test.

The beautiful promises may turn out to be on the side of over-enthusiasm. But let any woman try *not* using her share of those $7 billion moonbeams. She'll soon come out of the dark! It becomes more and more apparent that there is really nothing superficial about the connection between the way a woman feels and the way she looks.

Experiment "Lipstick Therapy" was tried at Camarillo State Hospital (for mentally disturbed girls). This was virtually a beauty and charm course in which the young girls were taught how to do their makeup, their hair, how to walk and exercise. Those who took the course left the institution in four months instead of the usual six.

Although the course was credited as *part* of the cure, it added a new dimension to therapy, as well as proving the whole woman-beauty mystique.

Improvement begins with consciousness of yourself. Make up your own beauty philosophy that suits you and nobody else. But have one. Make it your business to know what kind of skin and hair *you* have, and what you are doing *for,* not to them.

Don't buy something the salesgirl behind the cosmetics counter told you was "good." She'll say that about anything she's selling. And while the big cosmetic houses are supposed to be spending thousands, even millions, on training programs, it is a mystery what happens to all those trainees. Specialized cosmetics personnel seem to be disappearing along with all the sales people who, once upon a time, were supposed to know something about the merchandise they were selling. Even the girl who dabbed a tester spot of foundation that you were going to wear on your face on your hand, where the skin is altogether different, doesn't seem to be around any longer.

But never mind. It's an ill wind that blows no good, and this new forced self-service could be a better way. A sales person couldn't possibly know what suits you better than *you,* so it's your incentive to make it your business to know.

This takes experimentation, insight and some knowledge. Great beauties have made their own way to beauty a part of themselves. The mouth has an expression of appeal even without the lipstick. Now, in our unzipped world, every woman is a beauty who makes a beauty of herself.

The face is only an extension of the body, not something that functions on its own. To treat your body as if it weren't there is to be only aware of its shortcomings and pains, not its pleasures.

Of this *un*body consciousness someone put it that the body is the temple of the mind but the temple is in ruins.

Of body *consciousness,* there are do-it-yourself and do-it-for-you ways to go, or a combination of both.

There are do-it-for-you ways that are miraculously rewarding, except in the pocketbook. The fat farm, for instance, has become a part of our upper echelon of life. And it's a pretty cheeky name for an establishment that will charge you upwards (some of them *very* upwards) of $500 a week to get slimmed down—and after all, how much weight *can* you lose in a week?

Nevertheless, it's positively incredible how much these sybaritic spas do accomplish in a week. Or, in some cases, even two—if the client is *really* one of the richest women in the world.

It is next to witchcraft what they can do in the way of pampering both the body and the psyche into such a state of bliss that the effect lasts six months. Which is precisely how often the regulars go—every six months.

Between the massaging, exercising, beauty salon rituals in reverse (like getting your hair in condition, not backcombing it out of its mind), gourmet-type starvation and complete pampering, you come up with a final you that seems to result from sorcery.

One woman who had spent her first week at one of the posh fat farms said she "felt like silk." Whereas her usual state was to be as taut as a strung wire.

A lot of it has to do with its being a complete case of *supervised* pampering. And if you think it might become cloying to have every minute of your time worked out for you so you don't have to think at all,. it isn't so. Leaving the world behind and having nothing on the schedule but Project You is a certain physio-metabolic magic that has to be experienced to be understood.

Perhaps you haven't had the time or the wherewithal (translation: loot) to give yourself over to Elizabeth Arden's Maine Chance in Arizona (very snooty with Dior pajamas worn by "just us girls" as casual evening dress), or the Golden Door south of Los Angeles close to the Mexican border (what I think is the real class—casual quality) or to the Nieman-Marcus Greenhouse, near Dallas (a combination of both, Texas style).

I would say that if you can afford it at all—like, say, considering it a vacation—it's worth the expense, even once. You will learn a lifelong lesson in how to pamper the psyche along with the body—and some of it will never leave you.

It's expensive, but you will have learned what a silken tranquillity is. And you can always summon at least a little of it back because, after all, you've been there. Actually, it's something like having been to an over-age finishing school.

And when you stop to analyze what caused this delicious, next-to-Nirvana feeling in which you don't have a nerve in your body, you can see that the ingredients are available to you anywhere. At least the basics are anyway.

The tranquillity came from a complete waking up of your body—the marvelous masseuse and the exercise (which you did until you were sure you would drop, but you didn't, in as many as four sessions a day). While the circulation works, the nerves are eased. *That's* getting oxygenated.

Then there's the food that uncloys the body and produces a special clarity of mind. It is professionally prepared to seem positively gourmet—proving you can find 800 to 1,000 calories a day not only satisfying but a revelation.

And the rejuvenation of really leaving the world behind and not having to *contend* with anything. And lastly, the feeling that you are a superstar—but in private, with a specially designed privacy among other superstars—with none of the real stresses and strains of the real life superstar.

The last would hardly be good as a steady diet, but think what sheer soul-satisfying pampering of the ego it is as a special event!

Can you find time to slip into any part of this as a home routine? Too busy? Too many stresses and pressures? Are you really too busy to make up an agenda of regular exercise to keep your mind and body supple; food that you give some thought to; doing nice things for your skin and hair, and maybe even a regular splurge for the Sybarite, such as having a pedicure, or a life-giving thing such as a good massage?

I'll never think of a pedicure without realizing what it can mean, ever since I heard a little English secretary say soulfully, "I *lust* for a pedicure." She was working with a film company on location at Gstaad, Switzerland, and staying with the company at the Palace Hotel, one of Europe's poshest. And she summed it all up by the sheer luxe of the idea of having her toenails manicured!

Today, there are so many ways to the same end that you can choose those that meet your own condition. There are even a myriad ways to take a bath, if you will stop to consider the possibilities. Such possibilities have been a fascination since the Romans and long before.

There are hosings and paraffin baths and steam baths and sauna (for body and face) and seaweed baths and—what might seem ho-hum now—the old-fashioned mud baths. Some of these are being brought more and more right into the home, catching up with what used to be an uncommon luxury of the rich. Even if you don't have your own sauna or steam bath in *your* house, you can have a sauna facial and use it with an herbal mist.

You can join a good gym—and get into a regime. Women are too drastically afraid of weights, associating them with muscle. It takes a good long time to build a muscle into bulk, as any Mr. America will tell you. A muscle wants to express itself, to achieve a definition, whether you're male or female.

On the other hand, there's gentle, unstrenuous but completely pervasive yoga to be engaged in that affects not only the muscles but the being and can become a whole way of life. Yoga, of course, *is* a way of life.

Some yoga disciples, not teachers, just followers, claim that yoga changes the body chemistry to function so perfectly that they can eat what they want and the body maintains its proper weight.

Or you can discover that marvelous little masseuse whom you can go to (or she will come to you) and who can do more marvels for your body and your state of mind than you might have thought possible. Some of the success screen careers were first shaped by massage!

The point is, do *something*! Wake up your whole body, from head to toe. You can, you know. It starts by getting oxygen to every cell of that body—by *doing* something!

Thinking about what you are doing to and for yourself to create what you want to be reacts on more than just the way you look. It creates an inner-outer woman interlocking in harmony, as you were meant to be.

Even cosmetics, the good old standby stuff on the dressing table, seem to have become integrated with the woman herself, the fake one working with the real and becoming one.

Our era has made fakes frankly amusing, inventive put-ons, an extension and part of the scene of art nouveau and pop art and op art. Fakes can be artistic enhancements, measured only by the ingenuity of the faker. But what makes them valid is their takeoff on the real. There is more than meets the eye in those intriguing passion shadows created behind a fringe of false eyelashes. A girl may wear stunning eye makeup, but the face she puts it on has to be the real thing.

Hair has become a necessary accessory, not merely something you grow on your head. And what really makes it amusing is that fake hair, that used to be made from real hair, is becoming more and more synthetic, not real. The experts say that the hair you wear that isn't yours will soon all be made from synthetics, so it's a lot less trouble than real hair.

And *real* hair—the permanent kind that's on your head, if you're lucky—has never in human history been so totally beautiful. One more sex characteristic has been added to the female—sexy hair.

Natural hair has almost never grown in such vibrant colors, with such lustrous sheen and texture as it achieves today. If we seem to have a new type of *real* human hair, it's one more example of the real working with the artificial, so both become one, the chemically-created reality—inside or outside.

If you think that the modern masses of fake hair and layered eye makeup that Rubens would envy are something, the evolution of all gives promise of being far more involved with the use of makeup to create effects.

The woman of the twenty-first century may have a sheer, shining, blushing, luminous, frosty, or lustrous face—as the mood strikes her.

157

It may be in color, harking back to the classic Chinese theatre, where a face painted red symbolizes a good character, green represents evil, gold is reserved for gods and demons, both good and bad, and black means a determined will.

Symbolism in face color may be simplified by merely donning a mask. The combination of masquerade and reality will be part of the unlimited expression of the many levels of life tomorrow's woman will live on at once.

Glamor will play an even bigger part in her life, whether she is flying to another planet from a skyport, or doing her marketing and shopping from her space-vision computer at home. She will be able to push the button labelled "surprise," limited only by her own imagination, as Eve has never yet been able to do.

She will wear fabrics that respond to climate, expand, contract, loosen or cling. She may wear so little as to leave nothing to be guessed at, or wear nothing at all for swimming or sunning or wherever nothing at all is logical. Whatever she is wearing, the body will be nothing to be guessed at, and it will be the kind of body that meets such prevailing conditions with pride.

The art of beauty is a combination of the real and artifice, with one enhancing the other. And the best part of it is that the woman who combines them has to understand herself to achieve the result. It is one of the discoveries of self that the new woman is all about.

She changes the meaning of reality from something as it is, that she has no control over, to something she can create as she pleases.

Create your own beauty philosophy. Not just about makeup, but about your way of life—what kind of activity is yours, what you eat, how you feel and look as a coordinated woman. The means are available for you to be the woman you want to be. The ideal looked forward to through the ages is not in the future, but now.

Tomorrow is now.

CHAPTER 15

The Self Realization of Being Sexy

HAVE you stood on your head lately?

Or, to put it another way, do you feel that exercise is a dull chore and a great bore? Well, then, you haven't been standing on your head at all.

But you do agree that it *is* mandatory to get some form of exercise? Well, I know some women who have taken up yoga.

Somehow, yoga just isn't something you do with the idea of getting it over with, like taking a spoonful of medicine. There is something so precise and controlled about the ritual of yoga that doing it is like a special session of convening with the spirit through the body. You don't hurry something like that; you experience it.

It is one more of the Eastern means, new to our Western direction, which has been so long directed outward, in convening with the self. Yoga, as it has been said, reaches the intangible.

One woman I know simply stands on her head twice a day, morning and evening, for as long as she feels like it. (Standing on the head is, of course, a Yoga principle.)

And she lets it go at that. Her complexion is lovely, she feels fit and alert, she says her mind feels so refreshed it is as clear as a bell—and she is 72.

She swears it is all due to her daily head stand, which she has been doing for over 20 years. And it is true that reversing yourself like that for regular periods will certainly send your circulation up, up, and away.

It's almost natural for a person who does head stands to go into cartwheels, too. It really isn't too difficult to learn—but how many women do you know who can stand on their heads, much less flip into a cartwheel besides?

If you're inventive, there's really no end to what you can accomplish without boring yourself to tears. For instance, one famous star who hates exercise invented what she calls the "lazy-people exercise."

She just ties sandbags around her waist, wrists and ankles when she's moving about the house doing chores.

Actually, people have been using this "weighty" secret for some time. Now you can buy the belts that use the same principle in almost any drug store.

She simply discovered it for herself ahead of the horde—a prime example of the self-realization of doing something different, special, and your own.

It is taking a reluctant, but necessary task and making it part of your own thing, of accomplishing something in your own way. That is what is called style. And what has this to do with being sexy?

Just about everything. It was the same star who gave that famous Paris interview to a writer. It has become famous because she kept her hand in her boyfriend's lap for the entire interview, saying it made her feel warm and secure.

All the great *femmes fatales* of history have been great individualists. There was never anyone like them, before or after. For sex appeal, you could substitute personality—and mean almost the same thing. That's why their appeal wasn't based on looks or age.

Elizabeth the First of England was bald as a billiard ball under that red wig and she was in her sixties when she had one of the world's classic love affairs with the Earl of Essex, who was in his thirties.

Of course, she had him beheaded, but that was one of the privileges of Queenship. There is no doubt at all that she was a woman as well as a queen, even if she was not willing to gamble a kingdom for it. In retrospect, it makes her a greater woman that she did not.

An interesting woman can turn on a man a great deal more permanently than a flashing beauty, even a flashing *young* beauty. Looks may attract him at first, but he does require something more to hold him after that.

This is not to minimize the power of a pretty face. But it is also quite true what many an unpretty female has said out of sheer pique—a pretty face is not *everything*. It's something. It's a great deal, used properly. It's great for openers. But it is not everything.

I think I heard the best answer to that eternal question, What is Sex Appeal? given by a patient of mine. She is an actress, and the question came up during her appearance on one of those ubiquitous television talk shows. I heard her answer easily, "It's how you feel inside."

Do *you* feel sexy? This does not mean in the sense of feeling sexy at a certain time, or place or moment because you want to make love. It means, simply, do you feel *sexy*?

Do you give out vibrations? Does someone across the room catch sight of you and respond? That's not looks, it's your vibes working. It's an inner shine that puts the glow on you, regardless of whether your features are regular or not.

That's harmony, chemistry, personality, sex appeal. Whatever you want to call it, it means you've got something other people, namely the opposite sex, respond to.

Our own love generation thinks it's got dibs on vibes as its own discovery. Actually, this is a human electricity far more basic than their own concept of communicating by vibrations.

It is exactly what Rodgers and Hammerstein had in mind in that "One Enchanted Evening" when you saw that stranger across that crowded room. That's more than communication, it's physical.

When you've got the real thing, it's just naturally a part of how you walk and talk, act and react. It doesn't depend on anything you do consciously, because then it wouldn't be the same thing. It's, well, it's your own vibrations.

Sometimes the message is so strong that, as in the case of a girl I know, she transmits more than she means. She is just so naturally vibrant that it seems to become an invitation. She may be unconsciously kidding, but she is constantly finding that the receiver is kidding on the square. This much vibe can be embarrassing.

But what if your vibes aren't tuned in? It has been said of sex appeal that either you have it or you don't. Well, it starts, as the lady said on the TV show, with how you feel inside. And certainly you can become aware of *that*.

A current phrase, Miami-cum-Seventh Avenue-inspired, for not reacting is "a dead lox." Well, do you feel sexy inside, or do you feel more like a dead lox? (In case there's anybody around who doesn't know, lox is the Yiddishism for smoked salmon.) *Do* you feel sexy, or more like a dead lox? If the latter, just don't expect any counter-vibrations, because you're not giving out any to attract them.

Some women spend lots of money on trying to achieve those vibrations—clothes, beautifications, the myriad works that are at a female's disposal—and still wind up a dead lox. These women are depending on something artificial to create something *live*, and that doesn't make it. What they really need is a psyche-out, not a session at the beauty salon.

But then there are the other women who *are* brought out of their "loxdom" by these very same methods. They are the Cinderellas who only needed a little pampering, an awareness of themselves, to coax them into removing the dark glasses their real spirit was hiding behind. The external influence was not the reality but the catalyst.

Elizabeth Taylor puts a drop of perfume on her tongue. Can you think of anything further from "loxdom" than that?

Marshall McLuhan and his brilliant team at Fordham University writing in *Harper's Bazaar* of April, 1968, described this spirit as "a female [who] enjoys a lively internal sensibility." They enlarged on this aptly put inner ambience of women by adding that her attention was constantly being claimed by inner sensations, that her whole psychic life was involved physically. (Think that one over, loxes.)

Moreover, "she was always aware that her body was interposed between her inner self and the outer world; she devoted constant attention to it."

To go on: "Her body was firm, but filled with tremulous spirit. She created an impression of weakness. The erotic attraction she produced in man was not aroused by her body as her body, but by that mysterious spirit permeating it."

If you don't come already equipped with a built-in sense of this very real mystique, then you've got some catching up to do. Cultivate some clues in this inward direction; you may wind up turning on a laser beam inside you that you didn't know existed.

Do something to make you aware of your body, and wake up your whole body from head to toe.

"My great religion," said D. H. Lawrence, a writer who really understood vibes, "is a belief in the blood, the flesh, as being wiser than the intellect." What he was saying was: Listen to your senses.

The combination is both sight and insight. What you think about *you* is the essence. It is the vibrations that send out your message—hot or cold. How you feel about yourself is communicated in your walk, in your talk, how you do things, in everything about you.

Most of all, the inner psyche is clearly mirrored in the eye. If your eyes say something, because you feel something, you're already way ahead of the game.

Sometimes a glint in the eye will tell your opposite almost all he wants to know. Communication is not all confined to words, as our love generation has discovered, and shouldn't be. Who would be so dully pragmatic as to think so?

In regard to the male contradiction to the female, McLuhan expressed it, "In the literate world, the male ego has differed radically from the feminine ego in relation to the body. The male's inner sensations were vague, muffled. He forgot his body except in extreme pain or pleasure."

Again, the good old truism holds valiantly—*vive la difference*! If the male felt the same mystique about himself, the female would not produce this response in him to her own. The male is blunt, direct, searching, probing, the extrovert to the female introvert. Her psyche is complex; his simply says *now*.

An hour ago you might not have rated a second glance from him. You may even have repelled him. His memory is short. An hour ago was then. He is tuned completely to what is now. And if it surprises you that he can turn on as if he had never seen you before—try doing something to make him see you.

A male likes the thrill of discovery. And it doesn't matter what he might have been seeing right along. Not if he finds something new to discover. That's what he's really been looking for right along. (And therein may even lie the secret of why woman is the willing slave of ever-changing, fickle fashion.) We have come to regard the whole world as a happening. But it is better to *make* things happen.

The world is what *you* believe it is. You are what you believe you are. Tune in to that inner mystique—and turn on the world. Or whoever it is that may need turning on.

A beauty surgeon should know. That's where it all is: "Her whole psychic life was physically involved."

CHAPTER 16

The Smog of
the Subconscious

I DREW up alongside a police car in tied-up traffic—and the uniformed officer at the wheel was cursing, even as you and I, to himself. He was just as stymied, even as you and I, in one of those borderline jams in which everybody, from all four sides, has tried to beat the light. Left turns, right turns and straightaheads were in a snarl with no room to back up in and get untied.

When the snarl began to loosen up, he was the first to rev his car and shoot away with a zoom that let out his pent-up impatience. Even traffic officers find themselves in the same human predicament as the rest of us, without being able to do much about it.

When the frenetic, piled-up pace of life reached a pitch that affected the central nervous system as a screeching decibel affects the ear—Western civilization reached for the tranquillity of Eastern philosophy. From the incessant chatter of the mind we went to the relief of learning how to turn it off.

The unbearable ultimately must come to a solution. But some answers are so simple, so close at hand, that we miss them completely. Meditation has its uses and its users. But we might not even have to meditate if people simply faced each other as fellow human beings rather than antagonists.

The general selfishness rampant in our daily approach to routine living is appalling to contemplate. In our unbuttoned new world, the freedom of the individual becomes unthinking license. And in a world where there are more and more individuals, this becomes a state of screaming absurdity.

We are spending a larger and larger portion of our lives in our automobiles, and there are also more automobiles. Having to drive through traffic is not only a hangup, it is a traumatic experience. And it is the human element that makes it traumatic. Otherwise reasonable people, once they get behind the wheel of a car, join the cult of the manic driver. They release their frustrations along with the hand brake, and aim them along with the missile of destruction they are piloting.

Little solo psycho-dramas are part of driving a car. When you make remarks at or give those dirty looks to other drivers, you're actually shouting about what's eating *you*, not *their* ability as drivers—and you're sending your blood pressure up at the same time. This is the wrong side of the youth game. This is a bunch of little kids refusing to grow up.

When you lean on the horn first, instead of looking for the reason why that driver ahead is holding you up, it may even compound your own feeling of inadequacy when you find she's (let's conform to the prejudice and say it's a she) really not an idiot, but that her engine has stalled.

And what about those boulevard drivers who whizz down what they demand as their right of way and will kill you and themselves to prove it's theirs.

Not only do insurance rates go up somewhere in the vicinity of 200 percent, but the entire insurance system must be revised to meet the impossible situation. Once again, it's *genus Homo sapiens* who does it to himself.

What we do to ourselves on the highways and streets goes far beyond pocketbook and nervous system damage. We have lost more people in traffic accidents than in all our wars combined. Now there's a statistic that says something about the human condition.

166

There is some universal madness that exists between man and automobile. I don't know what the statistics are in other countries—but on the autobahn in Germany, the autostrada in Italy, even the M-I in England, where a civilized cool is normal—Europeans drive like they're on the Indianapolis Speedway. Japan, of course, is where only former Kamikaze pilots drive cars.

Nor is it only automobiles. It is apparent that we have a world in which we must come to terms with machinery.

While we are working toward ultimate solutions, what we need is a get-soft policy. Take it easy—and make allowances for the other fellow. Especially that 55-year-old man who is still defying his father when he cuts you off just short of a fender-bending, and then won't even give you so much as a look.

Tensions rise from underlying fears and anxieties. When you get yourself into a flurry because you are late for an appointment, it is not being late that gets you into a state. It is the anxiety, a psychological fear of the consequences of being late. It may even be a fear not directly connected with this appointment at all. Your being late has only triggered it and given it a reason to come to the surface.

Anxiety is the wrapping of fear. It is closer to the surface, so what we sense is the anxiety. But stop and analyze what the anxiety is about, and it may be, like the light turning off the darkness, that it vanishes.

Nervous fatigue, tension, anxiety, or just plain losing your marbles—they're all part of the modern condition. The condition is so prevalent that most of the time we are not even aware that we are wearing away our inner resources. It is so much a state of our being that tension has become the smog of the subconscious.

Tension can come from impersonal things; the street noises that envelop us, the contact with hordes of humanity, the constant contending—from the rude salesgirl, to the bad waitress, to the telephone operator who leaves you hanging at the end of a dead wire, to the unnecessary siren's shriek that murders sleep in the middle of the night.

Every time our ungodly siren of police car or ambulance or fire

167

engine assaults me, I think of the siren of Europe. It is just as persistent, but in what a different way! It is almost orchestrated, like a child's toy sounding off with adult humor. But it manages to be just as inexorable as the unmitigated shriek of our menacing, raw siren.

Add to these impersonal aggressions the personal ones that make our nerves twang like a toothache. The constant coping with competition, the pressure of getting the work done, the threats of insecurity, compounded by the fears inherent in a bewilderingly changing world.

Our life is a daily battle that begins with fighting the traffic and may end up with fighting the boss or your spouse, or even a thoughtless neighbor doing his share for noise pollution. And so the central nervous system revolts from the assault, and we become aggressive, high strung cases of nervous discomfort.

The pressures and irks that we live with daily are registering themselves on the subconscious part of the brain. And the price they ring up that we have to pay is a reaction of the body.

The mind and the emotions are just as subject to fatigue as the body; we know all too well how we sometimes wonder where that "tired feeling" comes from, when we haven't even been under any physical exertion at all.

The physical fatigue that comes from a good day's work or a day of recreation is entirely different—good fatigue, honest and enjoyable—because it is good to rest afterward. But when we feel tired and undone because the mind and spirit have reacted on the body to cause nervous fatigue, that's not good at all.

The physical results range from sleeplessness, rashes, migraine headaches, digestive upsets, to high blood pressure (whose other name, hypertension, is perfectly descriptive of what causes it). In fact, stresses produce everything from hives to asthma to ulcers. And such conditions, if repeated, can ultimately produce major disturbance of the glandular balance of the body itself.

Nor is this illness of our time, nervous fatigue, limited to any one stratum of society. It is like a psychic virus in the air and highly contagious. The stenographer who is jolted out of sleep when the morning alarm goes off is just as subject to it as the movie star who *knows* her hairdresser just isn't getting that hairdo right. And the hairdresser himself winds up a mass of quivering nerves, throwing his brush down in a pique. Nervous fatigue *is* contagious.

With women, this interaction of the mental and emotional on the physical self results in premature aging. Aside from what actual inner physical upsets may result, it is all too obvious that a pinched psyche shows up in your face just as plainly as a shoe that pinches makes you scowl.

You have always taken for granted that the archenemy of beauty is, of course, *time?* Not altogether. Enemy No. 1, who doesn't wait on time, is called nerves.

It is a mindless erosion of the spirit that brings on the set, hard, ugly impression of the face that no amount of "beauty work" will really erase.

That traffic tieup that ties *you* up in nervous knots, the words you let yourself have with an aggressive anybody, the strain of fitting too many things into too short a time, those nagging little worries you let jab at you—each one is a thief who steals beauty and leaves a calling card of ugliness.

The disappointment you didn't expect and react to with bitterness and tension can leave a worse wrinkle, a harder line, than time accomplishes.

And the general selfishness and ill will of the spirit—the antagonistic approach to others—leaves marks worse than all the others combined. There is no more unattractive face than the one with its fangs showing.

What is the remedy? It's a simple one, but like all the simple truths, a hard one to practice. Once learned, it can change your personality and your state of being.

How many people do you know who know how to relax? Can you name one, including yourself? First of all, relaxation is a state of mind. You can keep it even in the midst of the most harassing situation. A situation becomes what it is from the way *you* react to it—and never mind the wit who said that if you keep your head

169

while all around you are losing theirs, you just don't understand the situation. Nobody ever held onto their cool by giving in to the situation, no matter what it is.

There are many ways to relax: from taking a deep breath to restore your control, to setting aside an actual period of the day, or several periods, for being with yourself.

Being "too busy" is not a reason for not being able to do this. It is the busiest people in the world, those who achieve the most, who have learned how to relax.

No truer maxim was ever made than the one that, if you want something done, ask the busiest person you know to do it.

Although we are apt to think of relaxation as the art of doing nothing, we have to work to achieve it. First comes control—control of irritability, of impatience, of spleen-propelled reaction, of our instinct to take out our aggressions and shortcomings on others. Venting your spleen on others is definitely not the way to save yourself. A serene smile can do more to ease a situation than a whole court of mediators.

If life is a hassle, learn not to fight it. There is a man I know who, every time he gets into a situation that calls for flying nerves, thinks of the fable of the wind and the sun. It's amazing how many of my harassed patients I've recounted it to don't know this ancient fable of Aesop's. It concerns a traveler, walking along the road. The wind and the sun, observing him, must have had their thoughts on Las Vegas.

The wind said to the sun, "I will bet you I can make him take his coat off." And the sun answered, "Okay, you're on."

So first the wind put on his show, and he huffed and he puffed and he blew very cold. But the harder the wind blew, the tighter the traveler clutched his coat around him. And finally the wind ran out of breath, and he had to give up.

Then the sun came out and beamed on the traveler. The more he just sat there and beamed, the warmer and more pleasant the man began to feel. Soon, because he wanted to enjoy the warmth of the sun, he took his coat off.

Don't fight nerves with nerves. You can counteract them with a

170

little warmth. It's positively amazing how much friction could be saved if people just thought about that once in a while.

A good sense of humor is one of the greatest aids invented in the cause of relaxation. Humor and laughter go together. It is the sad, sallow people who find nothing to laugh about who also find their stomachs are as sour as their outlook.

Good humor is like fresh air. It stirs up the life forces to energy, stimulation, interest in the world. Again, we have a physical reaction following from a mental one. The stimulation is felt from better circulation, good respiration, the body functions working in harmony because the spirit is in harmony!

A feeling of humor and acceptance of what the day brings can't possibly include nervous tension. It is like an interlocking chain, reacting on others, making life better around you.

I like the attitude of the woman who had the unpleasant experience, as we all have, of being "told off" by a rude stranger. The woman just smiled in return and said, "Oh, I am so sorry." Her friend demanded, "Why did you let her talk to you like that?" "Because," answered the woman serenely, "to answer her, I would have had to bring myself down to her level."

Can you imagine a poised woman exchanging words with any-one, unless she were pretty certain of coming out ahead? What's more to the point, can you think of a poised woman as anything but serene, and in command of herself?

It is hardly an accident that she never arrives for an appointment in a nervous flurry, even if she is late. She is still poised enough to realize that getting into a tizzy over it can only make things worse.

There's another way—perhaps the best of all—to lose your tensions. People who are tense are wrapped up in themselves—they're worried about what they have to do and what's happening to them.

If you're not thinking about yourself, you can't very well be tense. With such exceptions, of course, as watching a suspense movie or an accident about to happen. But you'll fret less about yourself if you're thinking of others. Try meeting a situation from the *other* person's point of view. One of the most charming (and rare!) traits a human being can have is to think of the other person when the other person is doing the talking. Try it and see how lovely and *un*selfconscious a conversation can be.

Of course, if we had no "nerves" at all, we'd be at the opposite extreme: Casper Milquetoasts with no spark, no creativity, with an even calmness that had no peaks of excitement.

When we talk of "nerves" what we generally mean is people who haven't learned to live with and properly control nervous tension. One who is in control of his nervous system finds that a certain amount of tension is necessary and helpful—it is the spark that generates accomplishment, effort and peak performance.

We all know the tradition of the acting profession that if you are *not* nervous before you go on, something is wrong and you will not give a good performance. But that is *before* you go on. Even superstars admit they still feel those traditional butterflies in the stomach just before stepping on stage. But once they're on, the butterflies are forgotten. What remains is that "lift" that causes a supercharged performance.

This is *controlled* tension, as powerful as controlled horse power. But those who give away to tension, whose nerves run away with them and act destructively, are riding a runaway horse.

At various times we all ride this destructive runaway horse, but too many of us can't dismount. Being hung up and strung out may be accepted as our modern way of life, but it can hardly be called living.

There is an answer. Instead of batting against the unchangeable without, change the situation within. We must learn to make friends with our nerves and come to an understanding with our nervous systems.

Any person concerned with health and looks—and where is the one who isn't?—*must* begin right there. What good is it to eliminate the wrinkles by face lifting and then put them right back because of worries, fears, tensions, and harassments?

Even worse than what "nerves" do to your looks, the physical havoc they wreak makes them the prime reason for those overcrowded doctors' offices. Half the people filling doctors' waiting rooms wouldn't be there at all if it weren't for "nerves."

They cause a variety of symptoms from constant headaches—and migraine is nothing to speak of lightly—to a whole range of subtle, psychosomatic ills as individual and complex as the victim himself.

For example, I know a writer who periodically gets a pain in her right arm. It is so real that unconsciously, without even thinking about it, she begins to carry things—such as books and packages—in her *left* arm, although she is normally completely right handed. The pesky arm has been x-rayed, and the patient knows as well as her doctors that there is nothing wrong with her arm that a little peace of mind doesn't cure.

I am reminded of another writer who, even worse, gets a pain in his fingers from time to time. Of course, it is impossible to type and therefore to work then, since he is not conditioned to dictating.

Both of these people know that when the strain of work lets up, or sometimes just when anxieties let up, the pain miraculously disappears. Neither even thinks about such a thing as a pain *anywhere* when relaxing on a pleasant weekend. So much for the effect of our state of mind on our bodies!

Of course, the best known status symbol of our fast-paced life is the ulcer. It is the most common one because emotion is related very closely to digestion. And the ulcer is the particular ailment of digestion that stems directly from emotional imbalance.

The connection between the mental state and the physical ulcer is fairly well known: the stomach secretes hydrochloric acid that breaks down food to start the various processes that go into the elements of digestion. When you are full of tension bugs, the stomach is induced to secrete an oversupply of the hydrochloric acid. It eats away at part of the stomach wall or at the wall of the duodenum next to the stomach—the ulcer has a choice of where it will bore a hole.

The body reacts to outer as well as inner stimuli. When we come face to face with a sudden danger, the body sends an extra shot of

173

adrenalin coursing through us to cope with the foe. People have been known to meet such situations with strength they wouldn't believe they have, and normally don't. There is more than one such case on record of a woman lifting an automobile off a victim.

This is the body responding to an emergency with help by calling on reserve forces we don't even know we have until they are needed. This is the kind of tension that works *for* us.

But tension can also cause the body to strip a gear when the wrong elements are in the driver's seat. Adrenalin pouring through your body to cope with real danger is one thing. Raising your blood pressure at someone who has caused you an irritation, real or fancied, doesn't spur your body to action, it throws it out of gear.

When your emotions are out of control so is your body! How many times have you said, "I was so mad I was shaking all over"? Or gone through an anxiety feeling white and drained? Or been so "bugged" you lost control of your speech?

Fear and anxiety are the most destructive forces of living. Face the fear. Perhaps it is something you can do something about. Perhaps you are worrying about something either without reason or uselessly. In either case, when you look it in the face, you have taken the first step in coming to terms with it. A fear will either help you, because you have examined it and perhaps reached a necessary solution, or it will haunt you like a demon, because you have not.

Once I read an article called "The Gallows in My Garden." I was a teenager, and I have long since forgotten the author, but I have never forgotten what he wrote. What he said, in effect, was that the things he worried about somehow never materialized, after all. We all have a gallows in our garden. And mostly we find that it hasn't been waiting to hang us after all. The gallows in our garden is the fears we carry with us that never materialize.

Strangely enough, one of the busiest young men I know is also the calmest. And he spends very little time in his doctor's office, because he doesn't need to. This young man carries a workload that would ordinarily require three assistants. Yet he does it all himself. I happen to know that it *is* quite a great deal of complicated work.

Curious about it myself, I asked him, "For heaven's sake, Henry, how do you do all that work by yourself?" His answer wasn't that he loved his work, or that he was dedicated to his clients (his business happens to be publicity).

Giving me a level look, he answered casually, "Why, I just do one thing at a time. Then I go on to the next one."

The secret is as simple as that. While concentrating on one thing, his mind isn't bedeviling him about all the *other* things waiting for him to do. Instead of chaos, he has calm. It's that elementary. *One thing at a time.*

This is obviously not meant for the sort of person who is so quick to say, "I've only got two hands," when in reality he isn't even using one of them efficiently.

Incidentally, one of the best doctors I ever knew was the busiest, too, and he worked on precisely the same principle. His waiting room was always crowded. Yet while a patient was in the office with him, he felt that the patient was the only one who mattered.

Each patient was an entity in himself to this doctor, and each got his turn. He didn't have to consult his records constantly or ask the patient the same questions over again. He just had the power of concentration to exclude everything else but this person while he was with him. One patient at a time, one thing at a time. What a tension-free use of concentration if we could all operate this way. Come to think of it—can you give me one good reason why we can't?

Then whatever happened to the good old psychological rule that it's good for you to blow your stack? Like all psychological "rules" that have been adopted by lay interpretation, this one is highly oversimplified. To follow a rule of thumb that it's good just to blow your stack whenever you feel like it would be not only a dangerous habit but a dangerous way of life.

There is already the constant danger of spontaneous combustion from the friction all around us. There is such a large population today that people seem to be constantly rubbing against each other's nerves, like parts of a machine rubbing against each other instead of working in smooth coordination.

And we all know it is better to use oil to counteract friction than to just let the rubbing parts wear each other down and have the machine break.

There is oil to ease human friction, too. If you have a righteous grievance, by all means air it—to the right person and at the right time. It would be unfair not to speak up, both for yourself and the party of the second part. Perhaps you'll find that the other person didn't even realize you felt the way you did until you said so, and wants nothing better than to set things right.

On the other hand, if you don't speak up at all, not only is there no chance to straighten out the grievance, but you're setting up a resentment inside yourself. And you know what happens when too much pressure builds up in a bottle. There's an explosion.

The point is to state your grievance as a reasonable person, not in a moment of uncontrolled anger. If you stop to consider first, perhaps you'll decide that you can't set the whole world right, after all, and that it really doesn't matter that much.

But it's dead certain that if you do "want to make something of it," you'll accomplish a great deal more with reason than with anger. Disciplining your "stack" not to blow isn't repression; it saves a great deal of friction.

This does not mean the passive acceptance of rudeness or viciousness or stupidity. If you can do something constructive about it, or if it *needs* to be dealt with, it would be a sin of omission not to do so. But you can waste a great deal of nervous energy dealing with other people's aggressions when you do not know exactly why and how you are doing it. And the best answer is rarely more aggression!

An example of a woman who has signed a non-aggression pact with herself is Dolores Del Rio. Thirty years ago, even *forty* years ago, she was as lovely as anyone Hollywood could claim as a star.

Orson Welles called her "the most beautiful woman in the world" and was reputed to be in love with her.

In 1943, Dolores left Hollywood to live again in her native Mexico. But she has remained a symbol of lasting youth. And she returns to Hollywood often enough to renew the legend of her beauty.

When she made "Cheyenne Autumn" a few years ago for John Ford, the five-foot-three Dolores weighed in at 117 pounds, and in her Indian costume and long black pigtails, you could have taken her for a teenager.

Her eyes are the same lovely clear-brewed coffee brown that they have always been, recalling something she once said herself: "So long as a woman has twinkles in her eyes, no man notices whether she has wrinkles under them."

But the face that the lovely eyes are set in is unlined and smooth. Although her beauty is itself a legend, legends have also sprung up as to how she maintains it. She has been said to sleep eighteen hours a day and subsist on a diet of roses and gardenias.

Dolores herself says, "I have heard the silly stories they tell about how I stay young. I am not self-conscious about age, and I don't mind trying to clear things up. As to sleep—I sleep just eight hours a day. Always enough, but never too much." Of the rest of the "magic" that keeps her so unbelievably youthful, she says it is a way of life, not a search for the impossible.

"Some of my friends live by desperately trying to hang on to youth. They are frightened—and the fear itself is what makes them old. Everyone must get older, and to worry about it is wasted energy.

"I used to be dreadfully shy and full of insecurity and doubts. At that time of my life I suffered anxiety over the smallest things. So I set about to find out what brought this about in me. If you are unhappy, don't look for the cause in anyone or anything but yourself."

One of the greatest elements of youth is interest in life. Dolores Del Rio attests to this when she says, "Many times publishers have

177

asked me to write the story of my life. But I am not interested in looking back. I only look forward to tomorrow. The past is good only as an instruction for how you will live tomorrow.

"And what I worry most about is making the most of each day, so that when I go to bed at night I can say to myself: I have learned something new; I didn't waste today. I try to talk to people, learn what they have to say . . . to read newspapers and books, new as well as old, so that I know what is happening as well as what has happened. It is through the mind that I can stay young. That is my real secret."

Perhaps the real secret of her lasting beauty is that Dolores Del Rio has learned serenity. Of the women she sees who spend their lives in a frantic effort to hold on to youth, she says, "If instead these women would be sensible enough to lie down quietly each day in the peace of their bedrooms they would arise more beautiful in face and more peaceful in spirit."

This is a magic formula that any women can practice. Some do it by the habit of a nap after lunch. Some will close their bedroom doors after coming home from a busy day with a career and shut out the day's stresses before dinner and the evening.

There are women who lie on slant boards (a very good investment, incidentally) at some time each day, reversing the circulation—thus re-energizing tissues and blood supply—and find their relaxation that way.

A program of relaxation—time with and by yourself—is something that should not be static, but fitted into your own way of life.

The big thing is to *relax*. That starts with making your mind an absolute blank. You can do it even by lying back in a chair, if there's no better way. One way to do it is to visualize a huge square of black velvet and lose yourself in it. When you have achieved this, you have turned off your mind. You are giving your spirit and emotions a bath, so they can be refreshed.

There is physical relaxation, too. One way to achieve this is to imagine you are a piece of string. If you can do that, you're relaxed! A more involved way is to begin at the toes and work upwards, letting the tension out of each part of your body in turn until you feel as relaxed as a piece of string.

To lie down and let your mind go on running a rat race isn't going to do you very much good. A tense mind produces a tense body. Just let go—start by turning off your mind, like dissolving into that square of black velvet.

The time before going to sleep should always be a relaxation. Actors and actresses have a special thing, that they have to "unwind" after a performance before they can even think of sleep. This means they have to come down to a calmer level from being geared up to the performance. Well, don't *you* have to unwind after a busy day?

Instead of a quick shower or bath and "falling" into bed, only to toss and turn because you haven't got rid of your tensions, why not really wash tension down the drain?

Instead of the hurry-hurry get clean method, why not really give in to the joys of bathing? They have been notorious through the ages, with some notorious beauties. But you don't need to hold court at the bath, as Marie Antoinette did, or be attended by handmaidens, as were the ladies of ancient Rome.

But you *can* turn on some soothing music (not the radio, not even FM, because even sans news and commercials there is still the voice of the announcer, to jolt you out of this self containment. The idea is to relax the mind, not to stimulate it).

You can fill the tub with warm water, as soothing as the music, and a cap of bath oil, or even just some drops of your favorite cologne. The bath oil is better, because it will soothe your skin, and with it, your nerves. As a matter of fact, you can take a lovely bath by adding a cupful or less of plain baking soda to the water. Your skin will feel as sweet as a baby's afterward. And what's more, no ring around the tub!

Put whatever you like in the tub, but make it a "special" ritual. Have a bath pillow, perhaps, to help give you the illusion of floating in the water as you lie there.

179

Which reminds me right here that my wife once walked through the bedroom muttering, "Oh, shoot, I can't take a bath, I don't have anything to put in the water."

While you're floating, you might do a complete job by letting your favorite skin cleanser or oil work on your face at the same time.

When you feel your muscles have actually relaxed, it's time to dry your body easily, gently, with a large, luxurious towel. Actually, can you think of a more satisfying way to make yourself ready for a refreshing night's sleep?

The male equivalent of relaxing sometimes points toward action rather than inertia and points out that he has more muscles that need using than a woman! Martin (Dean), Crosby (Bing) and Como (Perry) seem to have reached that entirely nerveless state by making golf a major part of their existence. Some men relax by their poker sessions, although poker certainly does nothing for them physically! But perhaps we should re-evaluate that phrase, "golf widow" if we want to evaluate what exercise, fresh air and concentration on something outside yourself have done for Martin, Crosby and Como!

My own game happens to be tennis. Perhaps there is some connection between the hand that holds the scalpel and the hand that holds the racquet in making for necessary relaxation. It becomes more than a game—a special dimension to your life!

You can relax anytime you have a moment to yourself. Like everything else, relaxation is a state of mind. And it begins with you.

Some very famous men and women claim they can get along on four hours sleep a night. It's true. Their secret is that they have the gift of being able to "cat nap": they can fall off to sleep any time they have a chance. That's one knack I'd like to learn myself.

Maybe you don't have the knack of taking a five-minute cat nap and coming out of it refreshed. But at no time in history has it been so necessary to be able to turn off the sounds from without and tune in to yourself. It works better than the lips-drawn-back-

180

over-bared-teeth plastic smile that some of the far-out chicks turn on as a defense mechanism against the world.

Your smile can be a real one of good will. See how much better you'll feel—and so will the one you're smiling at.

You'll both hang tough and stay loose.

CHAPTER 17

Inner Ecology

IT is meaningful that in our period of neo-existentialism, when nothing is supposed to exist emotionally but the present moment, that the West should become for the first time so deeply aware of the mystic religions of the East.

Om, the sound of Hinduism, has been heard throughout the land, and *guru* has become a common word in the language.

There are many different gurus (teachers of the meditation of being) and as many ways of approaching the mind-expanding self-awareness that they teach. This awareness has no bearing on the god you happen to believe in. It is a psychology of religion of which *you* are the center. In Eastern philosophy, that is to say the universe.

The vibration inside your skin is the same as the vibration of the universe. Concentrating on that vibration through meditation—or listening to the inner self—is to get with the fundamental energy of the universe. Or, as a guru might put it, to become *one* with.

If this is a bit exotic to Western concepts, there are a number of physiological truths that tie us in not only with the universe, but more immediately with the planet. Man is seventy percent water, and so is the planet. Many chemical components of sea water and human blood as well as the liquid part of the body cells are practically identical.

Yogic breathing exercises have demonstrably altered the chemistry of the nervous system. Brain waves, measured in therapy tests for the recording of dreams, differ from those in sleep. Brain waves have a measurable change during meditation, too, being shallower and more akin to sleep.

Dreams are problem-solving devices, if we could read them. The concentration of meditation is such that, making the breathing shallower, it allows the body to rest, accounting for the reason that one of the first things devotees of this new-to-the-West existential state claim for it that "it is so refreshing."

The purpose is to turn yourself off so you can tune yourself in. And since it has been described as "turning off the chatter that goes on inside your head," the "refreshing" part is undebatable.

Perhaps the best known of the gurus, the Maharishi Mahesh Yogi, assigns you your own secret *mantra* (Hindi words are adding color to the English language), which is your own word for use in meditation. Which led to a new opening gambit at Hollywood cocktail parties: "You tell me your *mantra* and I'll tell you mine."

The original furor over meditation, when it swept the West like a new fad, has quieted down. But if we are hearing less about it since it came on the horizon as a way of enhancing our sense of perception, the fact is that more and more people are making it part of their way of being.

If you haven't been to the Maharishi's Ashram at Rishikesh, the holy city on the Ganges, to get your own *mantra*, why don't you just try *Om*, the sound of the universal vibration?

Bringing up that sound from deep inside you makes you vibrate like a kettle drum. The heavy vibes make for a mystical reaction.

There have been many methods, even before the awareness of the Hindu philosophy, that seem to me to arrive at a similar result, even if they seem opposite to each other. The stream of consciousness, for example, depends on undirected thought, in which you let the unconscious bubble up and come to the surface, while meditation depends on no thought at all.

Yet both methods would seem to depressure the mind, and unless we have some release from the constant living within external pressures and drives and tensions, our minds become pressure cookers.

We are all part of the life force and energy; everything alive in the universe is part of this force and energy. Yet, instead of this totality of consciousness, we live under the hallucination that we are a separate entity inside a bag of skin.

When you wake up, how do you feel? How do you react to the brand new day? Does your mind jump right into the tasks ahead, already revving your motor so that you can't hear yourself think?

Then you aren't controlling the things that are happening to you; they are controlling you.

Don't jump out of bed as though you were late for an earthquake. If you must, set your alarm ten minutes earlier. Then if you must indeed have an alarm, turn it off with that dividend, the delicious little feeling that you can just *lie* there and luxuriate for a while.

That's the point, to take a few minutes to luxuriate in nothingness, not to think of *anything*. Not the unfinished quarrel you might have had with someone in the family last night, and that still has to be faced up to today, not the phone calls you are going to have to make, not that the plumber has to be called, not whether the dress you bought yesterday is right for you, not that unpleasant person at the office who seems to have it in for you. Ignore for the moment that problem you are supposed to have a solution for, the ungraceful remark you made at that cocktail party last Sunday, or the uneasy feeling that you talked too much at that meeting with an important client, or that it's just plain hell to get up every morning and start the same old grind.

Not allowing the pressure to build in your mind, because you are simply not thinking of the things that cause the pressures, is a calm you may not have a chance at for the rest of the day.

You drift along, luxuriantly curled up or stretched out, without a thought in your head, but something strange may happen. You may find yourself back at some incident in childhood, something you would never be able to bring up with conscious effort. Some relationship that is bothering you—with your spouse, your child, your boss—may suddenly take on a clearer perspective. And the tasks ahead of you for the day take on their proper perspective as tasks, not as battles to be fought.

We *do* live our lives as battlefields on which we are so frantically fighting that there is little chance to be what we are, to realize what we can be.

You cannot indulge in this stream of consciousness in bed while your mind is on a battlefield. To turn off the constant chatter in your head is to free the subconscious—to let the real meanings of life come out. A blank mind is a marvelous truth serum.

Hemingway once compared writing to an iceberg, in which seven-eighths of it is invisible below the surface. People are like that, too, using only an eighth of themselves, and the poorest, most superficial eighth, at that.

Creativity is still a mystery. We do not know what happens when a Beethoven composes a Ninth Symphony, or a Michelangelo sculpts a David.

But Mark Twain had part of the answer. When his wife asked him why he was just sitting there in the sun doing nothing and not at work, he replied, "Quiet, I *am* working." What he was doing was giving the creative force within him a chance to work. We cannot all have the gifts of a Mark Twain, but it is entirely possible that many a potential Mark Twain has been smothered by preoccupation with the externals that got between him and what he was capable of. And whether we are potential Mark Twains or not, each of us has a self that it is important to get with.

There is nothing startling or new in this concept—we just seem to have lost it. It was Jesus who said "The kingdom of heaven is within." He also said, "I am the Vine, you are the branches." This has been interpreted to mean that we are all God, or part of God. More pragmatically, it would certainly mean that the life force and energy within us is one with the life force that surrounds it.

186

The subconscious is a strange reservoir we have not yet plumbed, that is responsible for what we are and do, and that we are only just beginning to chart. In the twenty-first century, we shall know what the subconscious is, which means that we shall be able to control our actions. This may seem frightening, but it is just the contrary—it is liberation.

When man comes to understand himself, then Prometheus bound is unbound from the rock. To match soaring outward into space, there is a soaring inward to reach the same infinity that has no bonds of prejudice, human aggrandizement, hate, and all the other human destructions that have kept man from realizing mankind. That is when man will not only be compatible with himself but with nature, of which he is a part.

When we understand our motivations, man will be free. Who, for instance, could be a bigot, when it is commonly accepted that bigotry is only the stench of unreasoning fear? We already know—at least, those of us who are not hopeless morons know—that it is vitally necessary for the preservation of the human race that we accept each other.

Or that, as the flower children, who really went back to the Bible for it, claim—we must even love one another. We are so opposed to this concept that it was, and still is considered an upheaval in civilization.

We are approaching a closer relationship to each other as human beings, and that has its unsettling aspects, as has anything that deviates from the norm as we know it.

There are so many different things and events in our age, as we move toward the twenty-first century, that we do need, as Aldous Huxley foresaw, to become conscious of the ways of enhancing our senses of perception. Simply, it means to change our attitudes.

You begin *inside*. To realize that there is your own self, which countless people have gone through life without having the time or perception to discover. They were just born, lived and died—with not a single ripple to stir the surface of life. It is as if the energy that can cause a whirlpool in a stream of water was never summoned.

Someone has described life as a mysterious necessity to go on breathing. What an apt way of putting all that we have not known. And how much we are just getting to—in how we make breathing have meaning.

CHAPTER 18

It's Not Age,
It's Ignorance

MISS Mae West is still coming up with a lot more in her pithy maxims than meets the ear. About the continuing ferment on sex education in the schools, she meets a sticky wicket head on.

"Teach the children about health," says Mae, without moving a hand or a muscle, "and the sex will come after."

That might seem to be putting the cart before the horse for Mae West, who is past the mid-seventy mark. The truth is, she is one of the youngest people I know. And still getting to the heart of the matter in one Westian phrase.

Of course, when Mae speaks of "health" she does not mean deep breathing, knee bends, and drinking your orange juice.

When Mae says "health," she says *everything*. What she means is a vital force inside you that makes life worth living and is itself a magnet that attracts everything worthwhile to you. That's what, on the shady side of seventy, Miss Mae West has still got plenty of. And, while wondering why more others don't have it, she has managed to put her finger on one of the very good reasons why they don't.

189

Up to now, you have been brought up on the proposition that aging is simply a part of life, and that you might as well accept it gracefully (translation: give in to it) because there isn't very much to be done about it. Those diehards who put up a fight against giving in were considered silly birdbrains who weren't acting their age.

In fact, the so-called birdbrains had the right idea, but they didn't know where to get the weapons. The spirit was there, but it was mostly stabbing in the dark. You simply had to be lucky enough to have an indomitable amount of built-in E.S.P. to get anywhere in the battle against time.

There really hasn't been too much known about what constitutes the holding on to youth and beauty. The search has always been for the mysterious.

And what we have learned is so recent that much of it is not yet general knowledge. The woman who wants to stay young and vital and lovely can call upon the plastic surgeon's skills to improve her outward appearance. This in turn has its reflection in how she feels about herself. And she can change her attitudes. In finding all these means, she finds herself as well. *That* is the key to the youth-and-beauty secret.

That's what Mae meant when she said, "Teach the children about health," by which she didn't mean exactly, "be sure and drink your milk." Women in the past decade have become aware that there *are* means out there, somewhere, of staying young and fit. The means is knowledge, plus a state of mind and a way of life. When we have absorbed this long enough for it to become general, children will absorb it as a matter of course as they grow up. They will learn more about the body, and how to take care of it externally and internally, and all the rest of the knowledge that falls in line with it.

Already, the date on the birth certificate is not nearly as important as the image in the mirror. It is the basis of the total personality expansion we are just beginning. The search-for-youth-and-beauty *misterioso* of the ages is turning into our everyday reality. Mrs. William S. Paley, wife of the CBS board chairman, and one of the earliest glamorheads of the Beautiful People movement, once uttered the now classic remark, "A woman can't be too rich or too thin." Naturally, having *advantages* makes it a lot simpler to be glamorous. There is the world of travel, the $1,000-a-week health spas, the famous masseuse who keeps you in shape when you *are* in residence at home, the custom designed health and beauty rituals for you and you alone, the supervised exercise at the right salons, the experimental makeups with an expert until you've found the *real* you, the sessions with that fabulous wigmaker, the skin treatments with that terribly *in* wizard of the epidermis, the appointments with the couturier who really understands what your figure is asking for—and, ultimately, of course, the visit to the plastic surgeon for long time perfection.

This doesn't exactly sound like a beauty cult that is becoming an everyday reality. Everyday reality is not really Kounovsky's in New York, where Jacqueline Kennedy Onassis goes to her special exercise instructor, and Mme. Louis Arpels wears diamonds on her leotard (after all, her husband has so many of them).

The trick is not for the woman who can't make Kounovsky's to shrug it off with, "Well, sure, *they* can do it," but to be aware that there is such a place and what it can accomplish. And adapt!

The thinking is not too essentially different for the woman who spends $100 for a Day of Beauty at Elizabeth Arden's, and the woman who takes the time in her mind and her day to acquire a little of the same by herself.

It's becoming a self-service world, anyway. The aware woman who shopped the designer departments *before* she bought in the ready-to-wear department knows that the $2,000 couturier original will be all over Fifth Avenue and the shopping centers in less than six months in the $39.50 adaptation.

Actually, we've even gone beyond that. It's no longer even the couturier original that means anything. It's what grooves that's important. And the grooviest is to make your own meaning.

The hothouse flower that took such pampering and care and pruning isn't with it any more anyway. It's even more important to look alive than to look glamorous. The frankly fake look reveals

191

more than it covers up, or it isn't the real thing at all. What it says is, "Look, I can have fun with this phony bag because what I've really got is for real."

The thing is, whatever the look, to look *alive*. Like you, not like some contrived glamor image. Jackie Onassis looks elegant in a kerchief tied under her chin. That's the action—style moves, like everything else.

The whole idea of youth is to be involved, and to care. The word "old" has no meaning compared with that. Chronology involves the past. What's happening is *right* now. Never before in the history of time has youth been so much a point of view, a seeing things as they are and, to coin a phrase, telling it as you see it.

As we approach the twenty-first century, we seem to have created a new time dimension, in which we are moving ahead like a rocket flight, so fast that we are actually levelling out.

We do not understand everything about time, but we do know that in an astral-oriented world time can be very relative.

And we do know that we could leave the earth for what could be a few hundred years in point of our time—but would be only a few years in space, so that we could return to earth centuries later in our time and be only a few years older.

With such ideas becoming part of our consciousness, it is possible that we can have a new concept of our earthbound time. You can even make time work for you, instead of against you. The old, eternal arch enemy can become an ally. Instead of the steady, thoughtless, careless erosion, you can put time to work for you in reverse. Instead of having lost it, you can gain it.

It's the same principle as, when we used to say, "If I had started that French course I was going to take last year, by now I would know some French."

Don't rue it, do it—and time will work for you, not against you. Only now it has revved up so fast that to start something is to be involved with it, to become part of it. Or better, it becomes part of you. There are no separate entities any more. Being "part of it" gives it a different meaning, or more, a total meaning.

The way to get involved is to make it on today's time clock. In our time telescope, instead of a new generation every ten years (and it used to be really longer than that) sociologists are saying that we are really getting a new generation every *five* years now. Anyway, that's their conclusion, whether it makes you giddy or not.

On the other hand, there is the wild preoccupation with the twenties and thirties, in which some of the *now* generation know more about the early Cagney and Bogart films than those who actually saw them in their era.

If you want to get right down to the nitty gritty, a case could be made out that the very young, who instigated the social revolution we are in, have a great deal more of an open mind than the elders who represent the Establishment and who are supposed to represent all the solid things of our society.

It was, in fact, the first time that the meaning of "morality" widened its circumscribed horizon from sexual behavior to the true sense of morality, values for humans to live by.

Suddenly, we had a world in which almost everything that had been considered bad taste by sophisticated standards became the bag to be in . . . it was cool to be hot . . . a violence of clashing colors . . . psychedelia . . . loud, loud, loud, everywhere that delivered the message and shut out everything else . . . the vvvvvvroooom of cycles in the street . . . hair, hair, hair everywhere . . . a sub-standard that substituted vinyl for leather and made it work . . . pop, op art that took not talent, but self expression . . . violence and flower power . . . violence and love beads . . . black light . . . flashing strobes to light our lives by . . . a philosophy that you could find circa 1954 in *The Alice B. Toklas Cook Book*, which is the most diverting such book ever written, and is also the story, during the twenties, of Gertrude Stein and her long-time companion Alice B. Toklas, the first modern hippies, and which cookbook was made into a motion picture by Warner Bros. under the wonderful title of *I Love You, Alice B. Toklas.*

And if you don't think a cookbook can be *all* the way out, have a look at the recipe on page 273 for "Haschich Fudge." It is preceded by a lively account of the salutory effect of eating the fudge, one of the recipe ingredients being "a bunch of *cannabis sativa.*"

This is the Latin name for a certain form of grass, the like of which is not supposed to be a standard item on your pantry shelf.

If you can read such a recipe, along with all the truly authentic quality of French food and of those two expatriates living in France and reacting very much like our present day hippies, and find pleasure and fun in it, along with a bit of wisdom, then maybe you're all right for this strange new world—and you don't have to be too alarmed.

If your mind is screwed up tight against letting go of anything you have accepted before, then you do have a great deal to be alarmed about. Our inner lives are so integrated with our outer lives since McLuhan told us that the medium *is* the message, that we just about *have* to become part of what's happening around us. It is hard to accept change if it is thrust upon you, rather than the other way around. Adaptation is a sign of flexibility and youth; inflexibility and unyieldingness being a sign of age that has outlived its time.

This reminds me of the old saw, "I am too old to change." Linus, of that lovable "Peanuts" gang is very young, and needs a security blanket against the forces of living that threaten him.

Adapting isn't really a question of age, but of being. If your responses have hardening of the arteries, too, then you're going to be the one to say "I am too old to change." At least try to understand, and it may bring about change.

When the space age became a reality, it was an earth-shaking fact that man had penetrated space to set foot on an astral world other than his own. It shook up the whole conception of the universe and our place in it. Earthlings had really to think about and accept the idea that ours is *not* the only universe, but that billions of galaxies lie beyond, out there in infinity, that are almost identical to ours.

194

Such knowledge had to change our thinking, our values, and ourselves. It was One Giant Step not only *for* mankind, but in the continuing history of the evolution of man as well.

Some truths are eternal, and will remain so. There were others that were truths only so long as they were useful, and we discard them when they no longer have validity. Not to try to understand this is to say that humanity is fixed in time and space for eternity, for better or for worse, with no evolution or development of mankind.

What has all this to do with not aging? Everything. It's like what I heard a young girl in her twenties say about it when the whole older-than-thirty generation seemed in imminent danger of being wiped out, "You don't have to be young. You just have to be with it." That was a revolutionary statement to make in the dawn of the youth movement—every bit of ten years or so ago.

We've come a long way since then. The young may have changed the world in spite of hell and high water, but because there is a mutuality in living, their problems are *our* problems, everybody's problems.

Buckminster Fuller, more than anyone in this generation, speaks for the world of the twenty-first century, and he is in his late seventies.

And I might repeat that Miss Mae West is one of the youngest people I know. Twenty-seven years after she left the screen, she came back to do one of the most controversial films of a permissive film era, *Myra Breckinridge*, and most of the controversy came from what was noted as the Geritol Set.

You never think of the word "old" or even "ageless" in connection with Mae West when you come to know her, or even to meet her once.

The youngest thing about her is the eyes. They are a serene and guileless blue-grey, a girl's eyes, but with a focused intelligence. An established Broadway star at the end of World War I, Mae claims she grew up in what she calls the "Belasco tradition"—David Belasco being the great entrepreneur of that era who believed stars should not shatter the illusions held by the public by being seen off stage.

What accounts for her sudden gregariousness?

She will tell you, "It's the young people. You have to pay attention to this."

A whole new generation dicovered Mae West on television, even before *Myra*, on the Late Show, or even the afternoon or the morning show—and they let her know about it.

One day her doorbell rang and there stood two young fellows from Kansas City. They had hitchhiked to Hollywood to see her. And they gave her a diamond heart on a gold chain for a present.

"Ummmmmmm," said Mae, "I got diamonds from the other generation, but this is really a gas."

The fact is that this is the put-on generation and Mae is the fabulous put-on of this or any generation.

What makes a contemporary human being? Being yourself—within the framework of the world you're living in! That's the quality that has no age label. In the end, it is the things we don't do, rather than the things we do, that we come to regret.

Yet there are still human beings so ill-informed or so non-informed about themselves that they don't know how they got to be what they are, what makes them what they are, or how they can control it within themselves.

Age too often is not the mellowing it should be, but a rotting. The impetus of the age itself is changing all that, despite our own age-old personal ignorance.

CHAPTER 19

Pill POWer

WE think about the twenty-first century in terms of the managed mind, of the biochemically managed personality. But because man will use machines to change his life into something heretofore only visualized in science fiction, does not mean that he himself will become a robot.

Man will, *must*, learn to manage machines, as he will learn, the more he learns of himself, to manage himself. That is the meaning of his true and ultimate freedom, if there is to be an ultimate.

It is something like working his way through different layers of evolution, emerging a little farther with each one—*its* frightening possibilities to ponder.

Machines cannot think. Men can. They must depend on men to build them, and then for the stimuli to trigger their incredible computerizations.

Man will have many ways to realize himself in the next century. The *inner* trip—going some place psychically instead of physically —has become the controversial reality of *this* century.

We cannot accept the belief that reality is entirely outside ourselves. We must acknowledge that it is inside as well. Twenty-five hundred years after the early Greek logic, we come back from the essence of pure reason to the concept of a reality within oneself, as well as the reality of the outward world, and that the search for truth has become an inward trip.

It is possible that this ultimate truth began to come back to us on the analyst's couch. The inner quest became expanded with drugs, the knowledge of LSD, and its new dimensions for the mind. Reality was no longer something to be observed, noted, and measured outside the person.

The ways of the inner quest expanded. In a Western world so filled with shock waves that it seems sometimes in imminent danger of exploding, suddenly there is an attempt to retreat into total tranquility—the means to be found in philosophies older than the Greeks'.

Some of us are discovering that meditation can even replace the mind-expanding drugs. Indian mysticism replaces the need for pharmacological hypnotism.

The turned-on chick who now seems to live with all her nerves outside her is a new breed of human being. She doesn't have the ordinary hangups of civilization as they were known before her. She may find others, but she has probed levels never known before—because she had to. In the retreat from the unbearable, she found different values, a different world to live *in*, not *by*, and her own *new* set of hangups.

Pills, the pharmacological, will have a great deal to do with the twenty-first century simply because we shall know so much more about pharmacology, and what it can do to the human organism, body and brain.

Pills will not be used to sinister effect, to create creatures from an old monster movie. They will simply have enough meaning to change our lives, even the past meanings of our minds. But without the fragmented, mind blowing results of the too-much, too-soon experimental excursions of the individual.

We have already seen evidence of this in the first major change-over pill of our human existence—The Pill.

The birth control pill profoundly changed our conventions, our mores, our concept of sex—and some form of it will eventually affect our population.

Then the safety controversy over what was the great sex liberator made it seem like only a pipe dream, after all. There are experiments going on now that are expected to make taking The Pill a matter of course, with no questions. It may take a new form, but Dr. Alan Guttmacher, president of the Planned Parenthood Association, has said that "the pill is the greatest invention since the wheel."

What it has already done is to pave the way to accepted birth control in various ways, and for both sexes. The vasectomy for the male is becoming an easy, common and certainly sure way of birth control. The female's methods of not becoming pregnant are between her and her doctor, whatever is best suited to her.

Sex is a human act as well as a procreative one, with biological and emotional meanings aside from birth. To be able to separate the two, for the first time in man's history on earth, is a virtual reversal of the man-woman experience on earth, if not in the act itself, in the meanings for each. If woman has been Prometheus-bound to the rock of her role as birth-giver, each man has had to come to terms with his own liberation in his role.

The ultimate possibility—that nobody gets pregnant—has become a great common denominator of the man-woman relationship.

In this new equation of the sexes, we have had suddenly to search for new values, new meanings, new justifications and even new truths. The age-old established conventions suddenly were under the fire of some new questions or, at least, questions that could be asked at last. Morality became a matter of adjustment.

But there is always the human equation. Liberation needs some moorings somewhere, and eventually finds them. But with liberty comes the freedom to make true valuations and live by them.

The power of The Pill or of foolproof birth control may eventually change even the status of marriage itself, although marriage has been changing of itself for the past few decades.

Yet the basic man-woman relationship, even if it is undergoing some drastic revisions, is an enduring one. Even if the sexes seem to be drawing together, as long as there *are* sexes—two of them—unisex is only part of the new semantics. And even if we really decided to grow babies in a test tube, even then it just doesn't seem feasible that man and women will want to give up the delight of the *difference* in each other.

The crux of the change is that a woman can be a woman and an individual at the same time. That has been her difficulty through the ages, and that's where the difficulty is now—in the adjustment to her widened boundaries.

"Woman's place is in the home" has been the underlying structure of our society, and that's where man wanted to keep her. Moreover, if she was smart, that's where she *wanted* to be. Because it was usually, in a high, very high percentage of the time, when she left home that she got into trouble. She either had to be very strong, very self-sufficient, or of a distinctly unusual caliber not to.

It was psychologically sound for woman to feel that her place *was* in the home. With the world geared to that concept, she had to be prepared to lead two lives if she attempted to do anything seriously outside it. Because then it fell to her to take care of both her outside job *and* the one at home.

It was only up to very recently that a woman who felt that she *had* to get out of the house was ailing in her psyche. There was really enough responsibility and aesthetic outlet waiting for her right there, providing she was happy in the acceptance of it. What she was escaping from was not the home, but the conditions in it.

Whenever I heard of the wife of a very wealthy man knocking herself out to get somewhere as an actress (especially as an actress!), or otherwise taking the tough road to personal success, I always wondered how long the marriage was going to last. In most cases, it was not very long.

Now, I am not apt to think that way at all. Could one revolutionary pill have caused this complete revolution of our *major* sex?

The answer is, yes, it would really seem so. Whatever form The

Pill takes in its current development, it has given woman, for the first time, the freedom to choose when she shall become pregnant, quite apart from its bearing on any other part of her life, including her sex life.

Together with this, the whole social structure of mother and home is changing along with everything else. Children no longer feel that mother was out there only to care for them alone. Mother is an individual, a human being, with all the needs and rights of a human being.

It may lead to fewer Oedipus complexes in the future, but it is surely leading to the fact that mother *is* a person, if we haven't been led there already.

It is becoming the norm for women to have a job or some other kind of interest, outside the home. It is, in fact, a rare woman today who doesn't. Even if she has enough time to use it for cultural development or the new directions of getting *involved*. The spirit of the age is involvement, and women are getting more involved by the minute. That magazine *did* keep telling us never to underestimate the power of a woman.

There is one other pill that has been playing a major part in woman's liberation *and* rejuvenation. It is the means for supplying women, biologically, with the essence of youth, hormones. By means of *this* pill she can go on being stronger, handsomer, fitter, more creative, younger—virtually indefinitely. And her own doctor can supply her with a prescription for this eternal liberation. Woman is no longer at the mercy of her ovaries, but has finally come into a world that changes the meaning of woman herself.

It is a far cry from the Soma pills of Aldous Huxley's *Brave New World*, in which the population lives in an eternal state of tranquilized nonentity. But it is a major indication of how pills will work to change ourselves and our lives. We know that right now laboratories can make up pills that will stimulate us to certain activities as needed, for optimal functioning. What follows is to understand fully their functioning in the nervous system as well.

The meaning of "drugs" will happily evolve from the nightmare of terror that indiscriminate use of drugs as we know them today

201

has caused. It has become an axiom that even in the superficially "straight" world, drugs have replaced alcohol as a form of diversion. This is one instance in which science was not yet ready for man, reversing the usual pattern. But it is catching up. In three to five years perhaps we will have the results, not the conjecture—of the shattering misuse.

In the twenty-first century we shall probably be able to take pills to change the color of our hair and the color of our skin (there is already one that can make us tan). Makeup may even be accomplished by the popping of a few pills for the occasion. And the possibilities go on from there. There will be drugs specifically focused to do only what we want them to do, to alter those symptoms we wish to alter, to increase communication and behavior, not diminish them. In the study of brain chemistry, scientists are even talking of pills to make us learn, of "smart" pills for our brain potentiality.

But one fact, so far, seems to have an inbuilt, strange sense of justice. Or retribution? Although women can look forward to an almost eternal youth with hormones—sadly, this does not apply to men.

Whatever *will* women do with all that *power?*

CHAPTER 20

The Marvelous New Unzipped World

> We cannot live only for ourselves. A thousand fibers connect us with our fellow-men; and along these sympathetic threads, our actions run as causes, and they come back to us as effects.
>
> Herman Melville

IT'S the liberation explosion—and everybody wants out. Liberated minds and liberated bodies, a freedom of action and a nude ideal, all adding up to a potential for fulfillment?

Or is it a moralistic breakdown of convention, a shattering of social bonds and a vanishing of conventional forms from the scene?

Of all the liberations, from the leg to Women's Lib, perhaps the most pertinent one is sex. Sex is a motivating force of life, you might even say the basis of life, and when there is a change in attitude toward sex there is a change in life itself.

The change ranges from whichever angle you see it. From a frankly accepted sex permissiveness, to claims of the die-hards who, in what seems like fond remembrance, say it wasn't really any different before, only *they* didn't talk about it. Even that's a healthy step forward, because it obviates the guilt that has always been associated with sex. But I don't think, even if I wasn't around, that it was quite the same then as now.

Motion pictures, that kinetic arbiter of our age, played a more integral part in the liberation of the body than Mary Quant and the mini skirt. After sitting through her first couple of movies that had nude scenes, one woman said, "You know, I can understand now for the first time how people can go to nudist camps. Why, nudity on film isn't embarrassing at all. It just seems perfectly natural."

This woman put it very well, in that in our social order we seem to have grown up thinking of the body as something *un*natural.

And sex, which is something private, becomes confused with something secret.

There is a dichotomy in our thoughts about sex. On the one hand, it is what the Puritan ethic has made it, with the artificially inspired interest in the forbidden and all its guilt associations. On the other hand, one of man's deepest and most natural preoccupations *is* with sex. As a human drive, there is none more powerful than the one for survival through progeny.

Sex is the most individual physical and emotional fulfillment in life, and it is inspired by a biological drive.

This natural irresistible force met the immovable object of the social order in the end result of sex, and the question had to be answered: What happens to the children? So the marriage-and-family basis of human living came into being in our society a long time ago, and sex became one of the privileges of marriage, and santioned only by it.

Even sex without the object of having children was sanctioned in marriage (with the exception, of course, of the Catholic Church). In fact, through the centuries, man has sought the sure contraceptive that would make sex possible without the end result of offspring.

Then, lo, in the twentieth century a little thing called The Pill came along—and for the first time in the history of man and woman, sex was separated from the accompanying corollary, and became an entity that could be praised for itself.

And in less than a decade the established social order was shaken at the roots. The pill was the greatest example of the evolution of ethics through circumstance to come along.

It caused the Catholic Church to examine inflexible concepts that its converts had lived by. The entire institution of marriage is getting a good hard look, if not an overhauling. And the people of the performing arts, always avant-garde, made it an accepted *fait accompli* to have children without marriage. So The Pill finally came full circle—creating a new conception of another kind!

One thing about that is sure now. There are no more bastards. Just babies.

Whatever freedom of action we have come to, I do not like the phrase "permissive sex." At best, it has the connotation of leaping into bed with whomever is handy, and at worst of copulating on meeting, like animals.

Sex, even liberated, isn't anything to be so wildly eclectic about. Sex is like nothing else in life, and is perhaps the ultimate experience of life. Since hardly anybody has offered an explanation of what the element of sex—the orgasm—is (except that it's pleasurable), it has something of the mystery of life itself.

Sex can sometimes be a sheer animal hunger, and it can sometimes be a great chemistry between two people in and of itself. But the whole human need is more than that, and it is most meaningful and enduring when it has something beyond that.

I think of the woman who approached it rather obliquely, but who had the right instinct, when she said, "You know, when I am having an affair—whether it's once or whatever—I am always a little in love with the guy."

Come to think of it, even animals have their erogenous zones. I have seen two lions showing their love by nuzzling each other fondly.

If they were playing, it was obviously love play. They were enjoying the human equivalent of necking—and what ever happened to *that*?—and very human they looked, too. Now we can shed one more of the old no-no labels on sex, that it is "animalistic." Actually, it's very humanistic.

With all the other hangups that we have lost in our thinking, there is one gain. We have at last come to admit that there is nothing wrong with *enjoying* sex.

205

But perhaps it is not all as permissive as we think. In Japan (and this is no put-on) there is a plastic surgeon who does thousands of little operations a year. It gives girls who are getting married a new hymen, in case they've lost theirs. In the marvels of our new age, even virginity can be replaced. But I'll take any kind of bet you never thought plastic surgery was capable of *that*.

A consciousness of sex naturally includes a consciousness of the body. So women began to wear a new kind of clothes that just seemed to go with a lot of skin.

The cult of the body calls for a new kind of "second skin" clothes over a free body, liberated from what had come to be considered necessary female contrivances to either disguise or contort femaleness. It is the cult of the natural, not geared to some ideal of what woman should be, but to what the woman *is*, herself.

Maybe it was Women's Lib that burned the bra as a liberation symbol, but it was fashion that took it off her first.

Mary Quant, or maybe it was Courreges, or both of them, freed women to an enjoyment of their bodies. And men to an enjoyment of looking at women. As one observer put it, "It's the greatest era for girl-watching in history."

In losing its age-old rule of the iron whim, the emphasis of fashion has gone from couture to detour, by way of Rue St. Honoré to the streets of the world. Carnaby Street and the King's Road and Via Veneto became the fashion happening of putting it on the way you felt.

Fashion became something not to put on, but to live by. The whole flipping world has become fashion conscious because our clothes are being recognized as part of ourselves, of our way of life, and how we relate to it. It's all part of the total statement about ourselves.

Again, the medium is the message, and what we relate to. Women tasting this kind of freedom are not likely to give it up. What could be more female than a maxi skirt with open buttons, or even a "see through" bottom?

But the picture is that of woman as she is, not as she was. Tights and tunic seem to belong to the world of geodesic domes and lunar modules. On the other hand, remembering Robin Hood and his ilk, there seems to be a human tie-in from the galactic age back to the middle ages at the same time.

Man takes part of himself with him, no matter where he goes, even into space. But he has never had so much fun conjecturing about just what he will find when he gets there.

"By the year 2,000, of course, everyone will be beautiful, nobody will be old." A young film and stage producer of the new international genre was talking. Actually, he is forty-three. Today, he is part of the creative vitality of the now generation, making the kind of film that is involved with its environment.

Only yesterday, against the new youth movement that seemed to be taking over in films, too, his age would have placed him as a bit into it. Since several of his films are famous for breaking the old mold of manufacturing movie moonbeams, it is a bit like the leader catching up with the followers.

The actual truth is that the generation gap is closing in, which would seem to be a slowing down as well as a speeding up process at the same time.

It's as if we have created a new time dimension for living. Instead of the old generation span, in the electronic world we seem to have a new generation every five years. There is the mass culture that says everyone has to move to his own rhythm, to be doing something that is emotionally satisfying.

Motion pictures, based on the physics of kinetic movement, is not merely the only new art form man has invented in 5,000 years—like art itself it expands the age.

From the conventional mold of showing each image in a succeeding frame, a series of images in motion on a multiple screen teaches the viewer to be selective. The viewer's eye is forced to choose, thus increasing his involvement.

The technique of diverse action at one time, converging on the same point at a given moment, shows the result in the action. The

207

linear movement of converging lines shows you what is going to happen on its way to happening.

Einstein explained it, in oversimplifying the theory of relativity: "It's like being up in a plane and watching two cars on their way to an accident."

It's the technique of involvement, and movies are developing it to the art of our time with the new shape of film. Images printed on 70 mm film (twice as big as used now), new types of imagery, hypnotic abstractions, are like looking through a window at something real that is happening.

All this may be a frustrating puzzlement to exponents of the Doris Day-Gary Grant genre, but there does seem to be a new audience for films, ready to experience movies in new ways, and equipped to receive oblique information. Sensory forms, not illusions, are becoming part of the reality of experience. Film is of the future, when we may receive most of our information kinetically.

Film is on the way to being part of our lives. Children learn the language of moving pictures on television before they are five, and at a not much older age are creating their own personal statements with film everywhere.

When the cassette film becomes a feasible reality, and that seems to be right now, then we will have home film libraries just as we have book and record libraries, and viewing films at home will come out of the exclusive confines of the Beverly Hills-Bel Air projection room circuit.

And even beyond that, the kinetic art itself is developing new forms. In August, 1970, in Russia the Institute of Cybernetics in Tbilisi, the capital of Georgia, held a preview.

There was no screen in the hall. A three-dimensional projection of moving objects, producing a complete illusion of moving characters, appeared not on a film screen, but in space.

The technique is based on a physical phenomenon known as holography, dealing with lensless optics, and made possible by the powerful source of light energy of the laser.

The connection between the concrete and the abstract once more? Instead of conjecture about the little green men who live on the asteroids, we find fascination enough in wondering about ourselves.

Will it really be true at last: Everybody will be beautiful, nobody will be old? In an era when life turns into science fiction, anything is possible, and a lot of it is certain.

Does that mean we can look forward to a future where we will all stop aging at twenty? I don't think so, although yesterday's far-fetched miracles do, of course, become today's realities.

For now, the mirror gives us the reflection. It is the reflection that becomes the image and the reality. The youthfulness of that reflection has been one of the closest things to human hearts throughout history.

It is the way of life *to* the future that beauty is no longer a means to an end, but an extension of the art of living.

If we listen to the right drummer, as Mr. Thoreau told us, the world is really a marvelous, unzipped brand-new place to get involved in.

In our own peculiar time telescope, when the meaning of life is now, not later, there are no marvels of tomorrow.

Tomorrow is already here.

CHAPTER 21

How Do I Choose My Plastic Surgeon and How Much Is It Likely to Cost?

PLASTIC surgery is an enigma, which is part of the fascination and preoccupation with its results. It is the essence of that spirit-reaching for the fountain of youth. No matter how much an accepted part of our life style it is becoming, that essence remains basic.

Although it is definitely surgery, it is not, and never will be, the same as having your gall bladder removed. The latter is purely physical. Cosmetic surgery is the combination of the psychic and the physical.

The modern approach to plastic surgery does have its pragmatic part. For one thing, along with the rest of medicine, it is no longer considered gauche of the doctor to discuss with the prospective patient costs and anything else that is relevant. And it is unwise of the patient not to have all such matters settled ahead of time.

What we understand, we do not fear. It is especially pertinent to plastic surgery that the patient go into it with a comfortable familiarity and—most of all—no lingering doubts about the situation, herself, himself, or the surgeon.

How *about* the surgeon? While the one who removes your appendix will do it successfully if he is competent, the plastic surgeon is, in essence, creating a new version of you. An appendix is an appendix, but one of the mysteries of creation is that each face is unique unto itself, and there are no two *exactly* alike. Not even with twins—or that mythical double we are all supposed to have somewhere in the world.

Perhaps that is why there is as much of an enigma in selecting the surgeon as in the surgery and the result. Again, unlike the surgeon who is going to remove your appendix, there is the added involvement of the psyche—in both patient and surgeon—that culminates in the result.

How *do* you get the plastic surgeon who is going to get the right result for you? One of the highly recommended ways is to see the results of his work. Or, in the same genre, but a much less reliable criterion, "by word of mouth." Somebody you know knows somebody who has had a marvelous result.

These are both plusses, but not to be accepted with the exactitude of a mathematical equation. In fact, anything that deals with the human equation is fallible and therefore never an absolute certainty. I have seen work from the same surgeon that restored one famous woman in her seventies to the veritable bloom of youth and left another with unmatched sides of her face from a face lift.

It is valid to say that it is wrong to even go into cosmetic surgery with any fear. Fear is negative. It is overcome by the much stronger, motivating spirit of hope. It is a beautiful thing to see, and I have yet to see a patient who did not have it!

How then do you choose a surgeon—and then believe in him? By starting with the facts.

One of the purposes of this book is to try to clarify some of the mystery of how to find a *good* plastic surgeon.

You start by saying "I want someone who is *Board* certified."

That means the Board of the American Society of Plastic and Reconstructive Surgeons—and none other. Your man must be, if not Board certified, at least, Board *eligible*. That means a young M.D. who has already had three years of general surgical training, plus two years of training in plastic surgery, but has perhaps not yet had the full two years of practice in plastic surgery necessary to be eligible to take the examinations to be certified by the Board of the American Society of Plastic and Reconstructive Surgeons.

If you phone the American Medical Association for names, they will simply give you the names of M.D.'s in your area who choose to practice plastic surgery.

So, if you are selecting your man this way—which incidentally, is a procedure recommended by the A.M.A.—be sure you make it clear that you are asking for a plastic surgeon who is either Board certified or Board eligible.

You can write directly to:

> Executive Director,
> The American Society of Plastic Surgeons
> 29 Madison Street, Suite 812
> Chicago, Illinois 60602

You will get the names of three men in your area or closest to where you live. Today, there are qualified plastic surgeons in almost all cities of sizable population.

Perhaps you should give yourself the benefit of seeing three surgeons before you make your choice. There will be a consultation fee (not commensurate with a plastic surgeon's *operating* time charges, which generally range from $500 to $800 an hour). It will probably be less than $50 for the consultation, and this sum is usually deducted from the surgeon's fee when you have made your choice. You can ask when you make the appointment.

Suppose you decide that all three men are qualified. Then how do you make your choice? By how you feel about a particular man. As I have already pointed out, there is something about the psychic-physical aspect of plastic surgery that requires a rapport between patient and surgeon.

213

If you don't feel this, keep looking until you do. When you do, put yourself in the hands of the doctor of your choice and don't hope for, but look forward to, the best!

Now you've got your man, what is it going to cost? That depends on you, the surgeon, and the kind of surgery he is going to do. The details are as personal and varied as the individual.

Prices vary from one part of the country to another and from one doctor to another. Sometimes (often!) they vary according to the circumstances of the individual.

General Price Scale for Standard Plastic Surgery

Face Lift
(rhytidectomy) — $750 to $1,500

Eyelids
(blepharoplasty) — $500 to $1,000

The Nose
(rhinoplasty) — $500 to $2,000

The Ears
(otoplasty) — $350 to $750

The Breasts
(mammaplasty)
Augmentation
(enlargement) — $500 to $1,500
plus the cost of the implant itself — $175 to $225
Reduction — $500 to $1,500
Uplift
(mastopexy, without implant) — $500 to $1,500
Subcutaneous mastectomy — $1,000 to $2,000

Body Surgery
(lipodystrophy—or fat deposits)
Stomach Lift: — $750 to $2,000
Buttocks Lift: — $750 to $2,000
Thigh Lift: — $750 to $1,500
Arm Lift: — $750 to $2,000

Hair Implant: $5 to $25 a plug
   Can run to 75 to 100 and even 1,000 plugs—10 to 100 plugs
   implanted at a single session

Forehead Lift $750 to $1,000
   (popular in Brazil, not standard here)

Raising Eyebrows $350 to $500

Chin Augmentation $200 to $500
   (correcting the receding chin)

Chin Reduction $1,000 to $1,500
   (pushing back the jutting of prognathous chin)

The Face Peel
   (chemosurgery) $500 to $1,000

Scars, Fractures and Related Reconstruction
   By the unit of time. A plastic surgeon's time charges run from
$500 to $800 an hour.

What about the hospital?
   Since some surgeons still will not operate anywhere but in a
hospital, and since we are still coming out from under the old
creed that the hospital is *de rigeur*, a good question. More, an
important one. It has been covered, as has most of the rest of this,
earlier on, but to get down to approximate figures:

   Depending on your surgeon (and the whole outlook on how
long and for what you will be in the hospital varies greatly with
him) the cost of your plastic surgery can be increased for the
hospital stay by an average of $250 (say, for a blepharoplasty or
having your ears pinned back) to $1,000 (the full face lift). That is
exclusive of operating room, medication and so forth.
   The operating-room cost is $100 an hour, portal to portal.
(That is, from the time you are taken from your room to the time
you are brought back from surgery.)
   Of course, even hospitals, like doctors, vary. And there are even

electives within the same hospital. Like flying, you can go first class or coach.

Does your medical insurance and hospitalization cover plastic surgery? There is no general rule. If your plastic surgery is done for health reasons—say, you have a deviated septum and in the course of correcting it your nose's outward semblance is improved too—then you might very well be covered. The best thing to do after surgical consultation would be to talk it over with your insurance agent or company.

Now—put on a happy face!

Index

217

219